# Recovering from Emotional Suffering

# RECOVERING FROM EMOTIONAL SUFFERING

## Current Psychodynamic Psychotherapy Told Through Eight Stories of Emotional Healing

**RONALD L. FUREDY, M.D.**

FOREST EDGE PRESS

 This book is not intended to be a substitute for medical advice. The reader should consult with their medical doctor and psychotherapist in all matters related to their physical and emotional health. To protect confidentiality, all identifying and personal information has been altered for all individuals presented in this book.

ISBN: 978-0-578-37254-9 (print)
ISBN: 978-0-578-37255-6 (eBook)
Library of Congress Control Number: 2022902767

Editor: Andrea D. Furedy
Cover photography: Ronald L. Furedy

First Edition
Forest Edge Press

Printed in the United States of America

*To Mother and Pop,*
*with love and gratitude*

# CONTENTS

# ACKNOWLEDGEMENTS

FIRST AND FOREMOST, I must thank my wife, Andrea Furedy, who encouraged me when I doubted the value of my writing. As a former technical writer, she has a talent for helping professionals who struggle with expressing, in writing, their thinking within their area of expertise. Andrea served over eighteen years on the Seattle Psychoanalytic Society and Institute Board of Directors as a board member and officer. Her ongoing interest in learning about psychoanalytic concepts was invaluable throughout the writing process of this book.

I also thank Russell Hicks, M.D., my friend, and psychiatric colleague, who read my early manuscript, encouraged me, and made relevant recommendations. Russ organizes an ongoing virtual group meeting of psychiatrists from my medical school class, a group of wise, experienced clinicians. I know our recent discussions are woven into the fabric of this book.

If there had been no Seattle Psychoanalytic Society and Institute, I would not have become a psychoanalyst. Nor would I have had the opportunity to learn from my instructors, my analyst Lawrence Schwartz, M.D., my supervisor and friend Roger Eddy, M.D., and my theoretically creative colleagues and friends. The eventual lack of one overarching psychoanalytic theory freed up and facilitated my widening development as a psychiatrist and psychoanalyst. Additionally, the greater analytic community in Seattle has been of great benefit to me in stimulating my exploration of many ideas regarding the structure of the mind, the psychodynamic process, and the relevance of contributions from many disciplines.

Finally, the decade I spent meeting with study group three from the Center for Advanced Psychoanalytic Studies provided me with in-depth exposure to the thinking and clinical practice of learned psychoanalysts from different psychoanalytic institutes throughout the United States. I am grateful for the time spent with each of these gifted analysts.

# PREFACE

ALL INDIVIDUALS IN THIS BOOK have been in treatment with me. I chose these individuals because they struggled with common painful emotional conflicts. I have modified and disguised all their identifying data and personal and professional history.

So how to write a book about psychodynamic psychotherapy while modifying all identifying information? The symptoms and the underlying emotional conflicts with the individual adaptations are accurately described, as is the therapeutic process and the use of other therapeutic modalities when required.

It is important to the professional field and to those seeking treatment for themselves or someone they love, to be able to read about and gain some understanding of the psychodynamic therapeutic process, combined with other treatment modalities when needed.

Writing, putting our thinking and experience into print, is essential for educating the public, helping individuals with emotional suffering, and the people who love them. There is so much confusion as to what type of treatment will help. I hope to convey to you my conclusions after fifty years of studying, providing, and teaching psychiatry, psychodynamic psychotherapy, and psychoanalysis. My hope is this book will help clarify the principles and practices that provide the best chance for individuals struggling with emotional suffering to have a clearer idea of the types of treatment they should seek. I also hope those of you who are considering pursuing a career as a mental health clinician will gain some guidance as to the type of training which will best prepare you for understanding this complex, exciting, and rewarding profession.

Ronald L. Furedy, M.D.

# Chapter One:
# THE BEGINNING

MY LONG JOURNEY of becoming and being a psychiatrist and psychoanalyst began early. As a teenager, I had a not too-well-formed idea that I wanted to be a psychiatrist or a psychologist. I knew I wanted to understand if anything could be done to help individuals suffer less emotionally and live a more fulfilling life. At the University of California, Los Angeles (UCLA), I majored in psychology and took pre-med classes. I was fascinated by the ongoing question of, "What the hell is going on in that person's mind?" I have been pursuing this question most of my life and continue to do so. I have studied psychology, behavior modification, psychiatry, neurobiology, family therapy, and different theories of psychoanalysis.

My wish is to share my experiences and the conclusions I have drawn, studying and working in these fields for greater than fifty years. Science will advance our understanding and clinical practice. Still, many of my conclusions, and those of my colleagues, are solid and will continue to represent the human condition with all of its complexities and permutations.

* * *

In 1964, at the age of twenty-two, I had just completed my first year of medical school at the University of Southern California (USC). USC offered grants to their medical students who wanted experience in academic research. That summer, I obtained a grant to participate in an ongoing research project associated with UCLA regarding the use of operant conditioning as a treatment for autistic children. Having earned my bachelor's degree in psychology, I was quite interested in participating in this study.

As a research assistant, I was expected to record the frequency of certain autistic behaviors: hands shaking, headbanging, walking on toes, social and emotional withdrawal, insistence on eating specific foods, and obsessively repeating certain patterns that had become very important to the child. The lead investigator believed that children were autistic because parents had positively reinforced these abnormal behaviors. He believed the treatment was to positively reinforce healthy behavior and negatively reinforce abnormal behavior. I was also expected to spend time with two autistic children, sort of in the role of a nanny. I spent considerable time with both children, just interacting and being with them.

At that time, there were three primary theories applied to the etiology of autism. The one just mentioned, and psychoanalytic theory addressing early childhood development, with maladaptation resulting in odd interpersonal behavior. Treatment, using the psychoanalytic model, was child psychoanalytic psychotherapy. This involved listening and playing with the child, and through interpretations, helping the child become aware of their unconscious emotional conflicts and defense mechanisms. In other words, making that which was unconscious now conscious.

A few investigators in the medical field were also exploring the possibility there might be abnormal neurobiology and genetic factors involved with autism.

I had no idea how to understand autism, but I did believe in the scientific method: empirical observations, statistical analysis of the frequencies of certain behaviors, researchers neutral to the outcome, and, hopefully, researchers objectively recording their observations. To this day, I still value the scientific method of double-blind interventions with a treatment method or medication, followed by patients and researchers, blind to the treatment methodology, leading to observational data that are statistically assessed for the efficacy of the method, and statistically demonstrating a low percentage possibility that the results are caused by chance or wishful thinking.

These conclusions must be validated by other researchers, using empirical research that documents the effectiveness of the treatment method. Long-term follow-up studies are also required to assess the lasting benefit of the treatment. Research in all areas, especially with psychotherapy, can only approximate these research ideals.

The research project I was on had some of these aspects, but the researchers were true believers, as was I, and this markedly distorted their capacity to be objective observers. The children were given candy if they behaved healthily, and voilà, their behavior was positively affected. This was documented, statistically validated via repetition, published in prestigious journals, and accepted as truth by many. Unfortunately, the study was massively flawed and there were not adequate long-term follow-up studies.

Sure, the children behaved better if you gave them candy after behaving in a compliant manner, but this did not prove that an autistic child became this way because their parents reinforced autistic behavior. Nor did it disprove that there are genetic, biological factors, or that the psychoanalysts were wrong in postulating that part of this could be causally connected to early childhood conflicts and adaptations.

Still, this study has been cited for the effectiveness of behavior modification in the treatment of autistic children; some value resulted from these investigations. Today, there are behavioral techniques that have some efficacy in treating autism, insomnia, obsessional thinking and behavior, compulsive eating disorders, managing children in classrooms, and developing interpersonal strategies for more adaptive relationships. These methods are not designed to explore or understand in-depth the human mind.

During this same research project, the psychiatric faculty at the UCLA Neuropsychiatric Institute decided to try a single dose of LSD on a few autistic children to see if this would positively affect these children. The idea was that altering the neurobiology of these children might have some therapeutic benefit. There was a commitment to the scientific method, and structured interviews and protocols were established. One child under my care, Billy, was given LSD. He was then placed in a room with subdued lighting and people were slowly introduced into the room, one by one. Billy did not respond to anyone, as was the case with the other autistic children. He just sat there as if the furniture was coming and going until I entered the room. Billy lit up and responded like an ordinary child. "Ronnie, Ronnie!" he called. He ran toward me, hugged me, sat on my lap, and wanted to play. No one, not my supervisor or staff, said anything to me following this event. No one noticed that something very important had occurred.

Decades later, I understood that Billy and I had formed a trusting, enjoyable attachment. For an autistic child capable of such an attachment, this has tremendous therapeutic potential. The evidence was right in front of us and no one noticed. I definitely did not understand. This experience has stayed with me, and, without being consciously aware of it, I have incorporated it into my understanding of an essential aspect of psychodynamic psychotherapy: If possible, form a trusting, affectionate attachment.

A number of empirical long-term studies in England, Israel, Germany, and the United States have all found compelling evidence to support the efficacy of psychodynamic psychotherapy in producing lasting changes. Healthy changes following behavior modification techniques tend to fade with time in comparison to the lasting effectiveness of psychodynamic psychotherapy. Many of the organizing concepts for this form of psychotherapy originated from the psychoanalytic literature and the decades of experience of psychotherapy clinicians. I am not saying that this treatment always works. We are not so lucky. What I am saying is that psychodynamic psychotherapy, combined with other treatment modalities when needed, if done skillfully, can result in a high percentage of individuals receiving a great benefit.

Throughout my summer breaks from medical school, I participated in research programs in alcoholism, psychosomatic disorders, and family therapy as applied to disturbed children. While I learned and gained experience, with hindsight, nothing influenced me quite as much as my experience with Billy.

A few years later, I was a medical intern on a rotation at a psychiatric outpatient clinic. During this rotation, I remember working with a teenage boy whose mother had just died of cancer. We met once a week for about three months until I rotated to another service. About a month after our final meeting, I passed this same teenage boy as we were both walking outside near the clinic. He smiled broadly and told me I had helped him, mainly because of who I am, a great, loving person who listened. I thanked him, felt confused, and a bit embarrassed.

I now understand that it was the relationship that was therapeutic for him. I was there for him, after the death of his mother. I listened and tried to understand what he was experiencing. This was of immense importance to him and helped him grieve the loss of his mother. He also discovered there could be other adults, and maybe friends, he could love and they could love him. From our work together, he discovered that loving was still worth the risk and that he possessed the capacity to love. Similar to Billy, this encounter resulted in my lifelong conviction: form a compassionate, confidential relationship, listen carefully, and try to help the patient understand their pain. Put words to their pain and understand the mechanisms they are using to avoid their pain. For this teenage boy, without being aware of it, he was emotionally withdrawing from himself and others. This rendered his grief more intense, but he did not understand. Together, we observed, put words to what we observed, and in the process, a bond of affection was formed. He was then able to risk forming new trusting, affectionate relationships.

* * *

In medical school, while working at the Los Angeles County Hospital, I was exposed to the horrific costs of psychotic disorders, addictions, suicide, and homicide. In the 1960s, little was understood. Medications were in their infancy. Freudian theory, while somewhat helpful in understanding myself, friends, and other neurotic individuals, was of little use in attempting to treat severe disorders. In essence, we knew so little.

As time passed, I became convinced psychological problems started early within the family. I took my residency in psychiatry at the University of Wisconsin, Madison, to study with Carl Whitaker, M.D., an early pioneer of family therapy. The program was wonderful. I was exposed to many theories, including systems theory, group therapy, existential theory, Rogerian theory, social psychology, and ethology. During this time, famed ethologist

Harry Harlow, Ph.D., was doing his research with rhesus monkeys. He demonstrated that physical comfort, when being fed, combined with the perception of a maternal object in early childhood, has a massive impact on the social adaptation of the rhesus monkey. This furthered my belief that the early childhood experience of family, especially with the mother and other caregivers, was core to understanding certain forms of emotional suffering.

We also studied Freud. I thought Freud's understanding of the difference between grief and melancholia, as being connected to ambivalent feelings and impulses toward the deceased, was correct. I also agreed that conflicts with aggressive, sexual, and loving impulses could lead to anxiety and depression.

After my residency, I left Madison for Seattle and was appointed the director of psychiatry at Harborview Medical Center. I believed in family systems theory and taught this to psychiatry residents. At Harborview Medical Center, like Los Angeles County Hospital, I was again immersed in human tragedy.

By 1971, there had been some advances in the use of psychotropic medication, and most of what I did was prescribe medication, teach medication management, and offer and teach crisis intervention. I learned a great deal and helped some people who were suffering. I also realized that the theories I had embraced during my family systems training, were not sufficient to heal most of these suffering individuals, whose recidivism rate was very high, and who never seemed able to engage in any type of available treatment when they were discharged from the hospital. Individuals suffering from schizophrenia, drug and alcohol addiction, post-traumatic stress disorder (PTSD), child and adult rape, and other traumas were usually not helped. They just moved along, frequently returning to our unit. Our knowledge was slim. How to relieve human suffering in such a vulnerable population remains a passionate quest for me.

After leaving Harborview, I moved to a community hospital and opened a clinical practice. I discovered the same suffering but encountered more individuals capable and willing to use psychotherapy. I also started attending a number of presentations by eminent psychoanalysts and concluded I still had much to learn. I decided to pursue psychoanalytic training. To be clear, psychoanalysis back in the 1970s and 1980s taught more than just the teachings of Sigmund Freud. With each decade, psychoanalytic training was becoming more multi-theoretical and more invested in childhood development. Some of Freud's original ideas were taught and still remain useful.

Early in my clinical practice, I worked with many individuals who could form a working alliance with me. Together, we explored their unique emotional suffering. Under these conditions, my ability to provide psychotherapy to individuals, couples, and families was possible. I continued to learn and felt some optimism about my capacity to help relieve human suffering.

# Chapter Two:
# MARY

TO GIVE YOU SOME IDEA of the type of work I was doing, still early in my professional development, I will tell you about my work with Mary.

When I first met Mary, she was a tall, attractive graduate student at a local college. She had just been admitted with suicidal ideation to the hospital where I was working. During her admission, she participated in group therapy, but revealed little about herself. She seemed anxious, upset, and hidden. The hospital was a safe place for her. She calmed down and then wanted to leave and declined outpatient treatment.

A few months later, she was admitted again following a suicide attempt, and she revealed how seriously depressed she was. While in the hospital, I suggested she start the antidepressant Prozac (she was later changed to the antidepressant Lexapro), and we began working together. After her discharge, we continued to meet once a week for psychotherapy. I was very worried, and I told her I was concerned that without therapy and medication, she might not survive. She agreed and continued with her weekly psychotherapy.

Early in her psychotherapy, she talked about her ongoing anxiety and whether she could trust her judgment. She said, "I feel anxious all the time, but especially when I'm doing my research. My professor is a good friend, and he is very supportive. Well… Actually… We are sexually involved, and I am uncomfortable around him.

"He didn't force himself on me. I agreed to the sex, but now I feel uncomfortable. I know I feel some guilt because I know it's wrong. Strangely, I feel taken advantage of. Like he forced himself on me, and he used his position to gain an advantage, but I don't think it's true. I know we broke the rules, but I actively pursued him. I don't know what the hell goes on with me. But I feel upset about it. And it's interfering with my being able to focus on my research. Doing well in graduate school means everything to me. I can't focus. I can't think. What is happening to me? My dissertation means everything to me, and if I am unable to do the work, concentrate and complete my dissertation, I probably won't survive. I'm so disorganized and anxious. I can't think."

I had thought her panic was the common intimidation that students experience at college when they are studying a new and complicated subject. I did not understand that she was unconsciously recreating with her professor, as she had done in the past, a sexualized wish to find the lost father looking for love and protection. Thankfully, I understood that I must listen, demonstrate empathic concern, and display no moral judgment or opinion.

A few sessions later, her mind wandered to memories of her first undergraduate year at a college in Chicago.

"I was all alone and knew no one. On the weekends, when the cafeteria was closed, I felt hungry, and I'd wander around downtown Chicago. I'd meet guys hoping they might buy me some food, maybe lunch or dinner. I had no money. My parents ignored me when I asked them to send money for the weekends so I could feed myself. My father was probably too drunk to do anything, and my mother was too angry. She probably just blamed me for running out of money, so I went out on my own. This never worked out well. The guys I met had no interest in feeding me. All they wanted was sex. They forced themselves on me. This happened a few times. I was so naïve and stupid. No food, just rape!"

The panic she was now describing was connected to her unconscious fear and shame of being brutalized and raped. She did not understand this, and neither did I. As with her time in Chicago, she had moved to the Seattle area to continue her education, only to find herself once again alone. She was seeking parental guidance and support. She was using her youth and sexual attractiveness to seek out help, care, and a way to not feel abandoned. Being unable to understand her actions, she felt terror, shame, and guilt. She also viewed herself as a failure. Fortunately, her professor was helpful in writing her thesis and did have a genuine concern for her, even though his sexual involvement was glaringly inappropriate.

Decades later, when she returned to deal with other issues, we were able to review and understand that the intensity of her terror and shame came from unconscious connections to past traumas. It is obvious, looking back, but it was early in my career and I did not understand the connection between present-day affect and past traumas.

* * *

Mary often talked about how her mother lavished continuous angry criticism on her. She also talked about how impaired and angry her father was, secondary to his alcoholism with daily massive, excessive drinking. Her father had lost his job, and her mother was furious and directed much of her anger towards her daughter. Mary left home at age sixteen. She was angry and wanted to escape the daily exposure to her parents' fighting, her father's drunkenness, and her mother's ongoing criticism of her.

Anxious to escape, she moved to Chicago and enrolled in a university. She talked about being unable to handle her demanding undergraduate studies; the emotional reality of being on her own; the lack of emotional and adequate financial support from her parents, and placing herself in dangerous situations with men. Eventually, she left the city and took off with her boyfriend. After a few months, she left him and went by herself to live in a very remote part of Canada. Again, she did not know that she had been traumatized by the emotional storms between her parents, their lack of parental awareness, and being raped. She did not understand moving to a very remote part of Canada was her attempt to escape the intense feelings she carried with her, as many traumatized individuals do.

While in Canada, she met her first husband, who, with hindsight, was struggling with PTSD from overwhelming experiences in the Vietnam War. He was kind and loving towards her. He was also unconsciously handling his PTSD terror by living in very remote areas and pursuing and participating in extreme adventures. This adaptation matched hers, but eventually, she realized that this was placing them both in serious danger. She was frightened by these wild adventures, decided to separate, and enrolled in a local college to resume her studies. Her husband did not understand her fear of dying and felt hurt. They eventually divorced. Decades later, his same counter-phobic behavior, secondary to his PTSD, led to his premature death.

After graduating from college, Mary moved to the Puget Sound area to pursue her graduate education. Unknown to her, she was still struggling with all the feelings that led her to escape to remote Canada. Unconsciously, she was re-experiencing her childhood and teenage traumas with anxiety, panic, and depression.

* * *

To better understand how unconscious memories can have such a profound impact, we must look at the brain. The brain has areas where traumatic experiences are stored and repressed. These memories are not available to the conscious prefrontal cortex of the brain. The intense overwhelming and, at times, life-threatening emotions are experienced by the patient, with no idea of what is happening. When feeling overwhelmed, we all look at our current day circumstances to explain to ourselves why we feel the way we do. In psychodynamic psychotherapy, the patient and the therapist together make other connections, once an understanding of the therapeutic process and a trusting working alliance are established.

When we are upset, and cannot explain it based on current circumstances, sometimes, if not frequently, what is being experienced is an emotional memory. This can be confusing. You feel overwhelmed on your way to work and draw the obvious conclusion that the feelings are caused by the work environment. Perhaps the overwhelming feelings are memories of earlier times when you were expected to perform by yourself or by others. The emotional nonverbal parts of your brain remembers and you are feeling it right at that moment. It makes sense when you conclude the cause of the feelings is work. This can, and frequently does, lead to phobic avoidance.

Feeling the feelings from both past and present disturbances, and continuing to feel the feelings while in psychotherapy, is an essential aspect of the therapeutic process. Repetition of these painful overwhelming feelings is essential to the working-through process. Repetition, repetition, until the cathartic process is completed, and the understanding of the complex interaction of past and present events are understood. This repetitious process is an important facet of psychodynamic psychotherapy.

* * *

Mary was likable, smart, honest, and engaged in our work together. During therapy, I listened with empathy and compassion. This was working, and she felt encouraged. She told me a friend had started attending Alcoholics Anonymous (AA) meetings and recommended this might be worth a try for her. I was clueless about her drinking. I now assume she did not mention it to me because she intellectually knew better and felt shame. She had studied the effects of alcohol on the brain. With her friend's recommendation, she found a way to address this serious symptom and avoid discussing it with me.

Once she had started AA, her shame lessened, and she revealed to me her immense daily consumption of alcohol to control her anxiety, and also as a way to have fun and sex. I clearly did not understand how she was using alcohol to self-medicate her panic, despair, loneliness, and anger. She was also using alcohol and unconsciously replicating her father's patterns and identifying with him, and as an unconscious attempt to be with him, not abandoned.

My experience with her taught me to be more aware of the possibility of alcohol or other drug usages that may stay hidden. She accepted my connecting her replicating her father's drinking pattern, partly as an unconscious way to feel connected to him, and to not feel so alone. She recognized that although alcohol had led to his early death, she did feel love for him and did miss him.

She objected to the religious aspects of AA since she was an atheist, but she continued and was able to eventually seek goodness as a goal. She decided that she was indeed an alcoholic and was going down her father's path. The path of an intelligent, educated man, who destroyed himself and damaged his family because of his alcohol addiction.

Eventually, she concluded that her research was not a good fit for her. She also came to understand that the driving force behind her academic pursuits was to discover why her father developed dementia and died in his fifties. I did explain to her the well-known toxic effect of alcohol on the brain associated with long-term abuse and how it will lead to death unless diagnosed early enough and treated. I had seen many alcoholics with brain damage leading to psychosis and dementia when I was a medical student at Los Angeles County Hospital. Maybe my speaking to my experience with the effect of alcohol on the brain might have addressed some of her confusion about her father's early death. Maybe yes, maybe no, but she did change her academic discipline to the same professional discipline as her father.

Mary changed her academic major and embraced political beliefs she understood as kind and compassionate. She obtained a Ph.D. in economics that allowed her to help people in need. She met her second husband, a kind, quiet man, and also a recovering alcoholic. She stopped psychotherapy after a number of years and went on to do well in her profession and have three children. I would hear from her now and then, and she was doing well.

One might say her therapy was an immense success and ask, "What more is there to learn?" I was using what I had learned: form a strong supportive relationship, listen carefully and try to understand, and work together to figure things out. All of this was and still is not only useful but essential. But there were emotional issues we never understood.

* * *

*Over four decades later,* she returned to therapy after she retired from a successful career and was in her late seventies. By then, my ongoing clinical experience and psychoanalytic training rendered me more knowledgeable about the unconscious mind of the individual. Over the years, she had retained a solid, trusting image of me in her mind, as did I of her. What we had accomplished remained in place. Again, this solidified my belief that psychodynamic psychotherapy, even when not completed, has staying power within the mind of the patient and therapist. Secondary to her maturation, my maturation, and the increased psychoanalytic knowledge in my profession, we resumed our work on her emotional conflicts.

* * *

She called my office and left a phone message asking for an appointment. I returned the call, and her husband answered. I had never met or talked to him before, yet it felt like we had a connection. He said that before he put his wife on the line, he wanted to tell me that her anger since retiring from work was difficult for him and her. He told me something had happened that he could not understand, but her anger was overwhelming. He then found her, put her on the phone, she and I chatted, and set up a time to meet.

By this time, her three children were all adults and engaged in different professions. Her daughter had joined her mother's profession. Her husband had worked for her company, and her two sons had started their own businesses in selling and owning real estate. One son used alcohol in excess. Both she and her husband were talking to him about his familial vulnerability to alcohol. She had sold her business and was financially secure. Her marriage was stable, and she had no major health problems. The last forty-plus years had gone quite well.

She lived about an hour's drive from my office. She had zero interest in having me refer her to a psychotherapist who was closer. She wanted to see me. She did not want to start over with someone else, even though it had been nearly forty years since we last met. We both remembered each other well, and we both felt an emotional connection. I was markedly impressed with how powerful the memories and feelings were in both of us.

For our first visit, she drove to my office, which was in my home, complained about the drive, and started to tell me what she was experiencing. I am almost immediately aware that I am in a room with a self-confident, educated, professional woman who is polite, and clearly, a force to be reckoned with. Where is the frightened young woman I worked with decades ago? How did she become so outspoken and articulate? I also notice she is about seventy pounds heavier, and I immediately start thinking about her health and wondering if she had replaced the alcohol addiction with a food addiction.

Looking directly at me, she says, "Well, you haven't gained any weight, as I have. Your hair is white and you look healthy."

I am thinking, but not saying, that she is assessing whether I still have the ability to practice as a physician. We both assess each other's health, given she is in her late seventies, as am I. I assume we both passed this initial evaluation since we began the therapeutic process. Not only were we evaluating each other, but we were also enjoying the reunion.

She starts talking about her company. "I sold my business to my colleague. She's making a mess of it. It's like she learned nothing from me. I agreed to work with her after I retired. Actually, I almost gave her the business. The agreement was that I would only be an advisor. I don't have the energy to do more. It's too stressful. I gave her the business with the agreement I would work in this restricted capacity only! She rescinded the agreement and insists I report directly to the board of directors. I told her no, this is not our agreement. She insisted, so I left. I'm so angry I can barely handle it. My husband says it's terrible to be around me because I'm so angry."

"You felt betrayed by her, especially since you had mentored her for years."

"I was betrayed."

She then spends the remainder of the session reviewing in great detail all the mistakes this woman has made. The intensity of her anger is difficult to sit with, and I assume this is her needed catharsis. Once again, my job is to listen and accept that she feels what she feels. My job is to provide a safe place for her to have and express her feelings; the more complicated understanding comes later.

* * *

As before, we agree to meet once a week, and she expects, like before, that this will probably be for the long haul.

At the next session, she continues to rant about what this woman has done to her and to the business she has built.

I decided to stay with the present events and say, "You spent decades building your business, and you almost gave it to her, with the only agreement that you would work in a more limited capacity. She backed away from this gift and agreement and you are understandably upset. Is it possible that she doesn't have the ability to manage the complexity of the business? Maybe she doesn't have all of your skills?"

"I never thought of that. I assumed she had learned all there was to learn. For God's sake, we've worked together for at least twenty-five years. How could she not know? My husband tells me I expect too much from people, including him. He tells me I'm too angry. I am angry, so much of the time."

* * *

The next two years are filled with strong emotional reactions to a combination of past and present events. We traverse emotional terrain from all phases of her life, including her beginning awareness that she is aging, developing some medical problems, orthopedic problems. Her mortality is no longer a concept for the future. She is seventy-eight, her father died in his fifties, her mother, who is in her nineties, needs assisted living, her brother, who is three years older, has just died, and within the next year, her mother will also die.

Health issues are becoming more problematic. She experiences pain when walking because of one hip, significant arthritis in a shoulder, and hypertension requiring medical treatment. Throughout the remainder of our work together, up to the point of my retirement, we talk about health issues. We also talk about her need to face her use of food to attempt to squash her intense feelings. She has no difficulty understanding the connection between her unhealthy uses of food as an addictive pattern similar to her past use of alcohol. She has remained abstinent from alcohol for the last forty years. She says, "I guess I couldn't handle my feelings when I was young and we were working together. I'm now doing something similar with food."

She addresses her hypertension with her family doctor. She makes arrangements with an orthopedic surgeon for an evaluation and eventually has corrective surgery on her painful shoulder. She puts an end to buying and storing food, mostly sweets, that triggers her addictive eating.

She loses most of the extra weight, exercises, and feels healthier. Why would she shift to a healthier attitude towards her health and her body when restarting therapy? She had been expressing her intense, helpless, angry, resentful disappointment by ignoring and neglecting her body. Within the safe and therapeutic space of our relationship, she finds her capacity to use her knowledge, experience, and her wish to continue to live and not be impaired.

In addition, she addresses her disappointment that her plans for her business to continue and thrive were not working. Her colleague was unable to keep the business open. A business she had spent over thirty years building was now gone.

There are so many disappointments that are a part of aging. No matter how professionally and financially successful you are, your body ages, the world doesn't change in the way you had hoped. Your family members are imperfect, and the time of your being alive is dwindling. I understood part of her anger was connected to the necessary grieving of aging. Life, yourself, others, your country, the universe, do not deliver the results one hopes for. We all endure significant loss and being able to grieve the reality of life, and how that does not measure up to our childhood and young adulthood expectations is not an easy aspect of the life we all traverse.

For Mary, at this time, it is more difficult than for most. Again, I conclude that she needs me to listen and attempt to understand. I also assume part of what will be found are again emotional connections to childhood and teenage traumas, combined with maladaptive defense mechanisms she uses to attempt to deal with her overwhelming feelings, like addictive eating and compulsive anger.

* * *

She starts the next session with annoyance and anger. "I'm the president of the homeowners' association and I'm establishing emergency contingency plans. Most of my neighbors show no interest or don't attend meetings. They don't bother to learn how to use the equipment. How do they expect to communicate and protect each other if they don't know how to use the equipment? I get so frustrated!"

"You took on the responsibility to organize this?"

"Yes, somebody must do it. What will happen to us if there are earthquakes, cyber-attacks, or any other danger to our community? They are so complacent as if none of this will ever happen."

"It's hard for you to accept that they are not as motivated and knowledgeable as you are."

"How can they not understand that emergencies happen? If we are not prepared, we will all suffer, we will not survive."

* * *

Around the time of the presidential election, she assumes a volunteer position for her political party in her legislative district to get out the vote. She chairs meetings and actively participates in phone and texting activities.

"I'm working with the progressives. I'm texting messages to get people to vote. I am also responding to those Republican diatribes about vaccine mandates and all that conservative crap. They say nasty things on Twitter. I get so angry. It is so clear that progressives care about the more vulnerable and the Republicans are all about money and avoiding taxes. I hate their attitude. I hate their capitalism. Why do they not understand that socialism is not an evil movement, but a movement of compassion? I just hate them."

"You are saying that you hate the millions of people in our country who are wary of change and feel safer if things remain as they were."

The session is on Zoom since we are deep into the COVID-19 pandemic. She abruptly ends the Zoom session. She hangs up on me.

* * *

In the next session, she apologizes for her action. "I had been dealing with all these right-wing political rants all day, and I just couldn't listen to your response."

"I think we are seeing that your anger is directed towards others who seem indifferent to preparing for potential danger, and those who disagree with you."

"Yeah, you're right. I can't stand ignorance, and maybe I am becoming more and more like my mother as I grow older. She was always angry at the failings of others. She came from a wealthy, prestigious family in Chicago. I've been going through her files about the history of our family. Her father, my grandfather, was quite the inventor and had local and some national acclaim. She was arrogant and went on and on about the shortcomings of people they knew. Shit! That does sound like me. I do have difficulty accepting lack of knowledge and ability in other people."

"In your work, you chose to protect the disadvantaged. You have developed quite a reputation in your community. Maybe this level of commitment and achievement was what your mother expected of you and now you expect it of yourself. When you, or others, don't meet these high standards, you identify with your mother's reaction and respond with anger and disdain."

"Did I tell you that I have been meeting with my colleague who took over my business? Even though she was closing down my business and doing less and less work, I wasn't angry. I could see there was just so much she did not understand. I was expecting way too much of her. My expectations went beyond her abilities. Still, it's such a disappointment to see a business I built from scratch dissolve into nothing."

"Yes, I can understand your disappointment."

* * *

One year after her brother's death, as he had requested, she made arrangements to scatter his ashes at a special place in the Cascade Range. She had been the primary family member who had visited him regularly in the nursing home, and he had appointed her the executor of his estate.

"I know he had been divorced for decades, and he was not close to his children, but his daughter and son could have made more of an attempt to visit him and be more involved in the ceremony. I am so angry with them for being irresponsible, showing no concern for him, and making no arrangements on their own. All they did was attend and witness the scattering of his ashes as he had requested. His divorce was an angry divorce, and my niece and nephew lived with their mother and had little contact with my brother. His illness prevented him from reaching out. He was bedbound for about a decade."

"It is sad, and hard to accept that the relationship between children and their parents can be damaged and maybe even lost. It is painful to accept."

"Yes, it is. Are you saying that I'm dealing with my disappointment and sadness by covering it with anger?"

* * *

The pandemic is in full bloom, and the state has masking, distancing, and ventilation requirements for all medical and physician offices. She wants to see me in person and gives long, angry explanations as to why those requirements are not necessary. I speak to my legal and moral responsibility to protect my patients and follow Washington State and the Centers for Disease Control and Prevention (CDC) guidelines.

I say, "With Zoom, we can easily see and hear each other. Since we would both need to be masked and distanced, I am concerned being able to see and hear each other might be more difficult."

"I am so angry with you. I meet with friends and family and we don't do any of that. It is not necessary."

At the next session, she says, "You're right, it is a state requirement for all medical offices. I volunteered at the hospital, and everybody was required to mask up and keep a distance. Why was I so upset with you? You are just doing your job, and legally you shouldn't violate the CDC guidelines. If anybody should understand that, it's me. Why was I so upset?"

"I think you took this as evidence that I didn't want to see you. You are feeling isolated and lonely at times, as am I, and at that moment, in the last session, your emotional mind experienced this as rejection, like I didn't want to see you."

* * *

A few weeks later, she talks about how well she is doing with keeping the sweets out of the house, and how she is physically feeling better. She is able to walk a few miles every day in her neighborhood. Now that she is working cooperatively with her family doctor and taking the medication and restricting her salt intake, her blood pressure is under good control.

She recognizes she is feeling less angry about the disappointments of life, her life in particular, and she is motivated to take better care of herself rather than being angry and saying to herself, "Screw it," and eating unhealthy foods. She knows she does not feel as angry and is more able to accept the reality of life and people.

* * *

The session starts, and she launches into her feelings of anger toward her husband.

"I am so angry with my husband. He has never initiated sex, and now, even when I do, he is not interested. I tried talking with him about it, and he said his penis doesn't work anymore. He is not interested in trying Cialis or seeing his doctor about this. He's about sixty pounds overweight and will not accept he has been eating addictively with me. He just had abdominal surgery to remove a benign tumor, and he has sleep apnea. But why is there no interest? He is only seventy-six. He's a few years younger than me. What type of man is he?"

"He's an older man in his seventies. That's the kind of man he is. You know he has some medical problems, and you know he has always been a bit sexually shy."

"I'm older than he is, and I still want sex. He will not look at pornography with me, read books, or try different things. What the hell is going on?"

"About seventy percent of men lose their ability to have or sustain an erection in their seventies. You have told me numerous times that you believe your husband has some avoidant personality traits. These traits have always been there. I think this is another example of you acting like your mother and being critical, rather than accepting your husband is now older. He has the personality he has, and his body no longer responds with an erection, which probably creates considerable embarrassment for him."

"Some older men are still sexual. Some explore other options. This is so disappointing. Why can't he be different?"

"I think you chose a quiet, dependable, not assertive man to marry. You have been with wild men. You chose a man well-suited to being a father, and being available to his children, and you."

"Yes, I know, but I still want it to be different. If it weren't for him, I would not have been able to obtain my Ph.D. in economics and also have children. He stayed home and took care of the children when I was in school, and when I was establishing my business. He would also work at my office. His writing skills and attention to detail were great. And he would leave in the afternoon when the kids were coming home from school so that they would not be all alone. He really came through. The other guys I dated or my ex-husband would never have done that. Why can't I be satisfied?"

"I think this is also another example of the difficulty you have in accepting the changes that occur as you and your husband age. It is difficult for everybody, but I think it is more difficult for you."

"Well, how so? I think I'm doing fine with aging. I'm now active, eating healthy foods, and seeing my doctor regularly. I stay busy. I'm still involved with my profession on a volunteer basis. How am I not accepting aging?"

"What you say is true, and many would cite you as an example of aging gracefully, but hidden in all the activities, there is a refusal."

"What type of refusal are you talking about? My great-aunt kept going to her social club until her death. She was almost 100 years old. She was active."

"Yes, but not anything like what you do. You exhaust yourself daily with volunteering at the hospital, at the board, at the clinic, at the political party, and on and on. You just agreed to be the volunteer director of the clinic. You told me that you had an angry meltdown at the auto dealership because it took an hour longer than you expected. You had an important professional meeting to attend, and you were outraged that the mechanics would interfere with your schedule. You are the least retired, retired person I know. You are scheduling yourself beyond your capacity. Your exhaustion is part of the reason you have these angry meltdowns. Many of us struggle against giving up our professional or business identity, but you are clearly over the top."

"Okay, you are correct. I've wondered why I make myself so busy. I volunteer for everything. I think it is how I feel okay about myself. Like if I'm helping others, I know I'm a good person. So, you are also saying I'm doing something similar with my husband by not accepting the changes in him. That I am expecting him to be someone he is not able to be. And when I see changes secondary to his aging, I feel like I'm getting even less than I had. I truly am difficult to please. I have difficulty being pleased with myself."

"It's like having your dissatisfied mother in your head, where you are almost always in danger of not measuring up to some ridiculously believed family standard."

"So, in my mind, I am always in danger of not meeting my mother's expectations, since she was never, ever satisfied."

* * *

Because of the COVID-19 pandemic, I extended my clinical practice retirement date by six months. I had been seeing all patients and students virtually, and the isolation and fear that we were all feeling made retiring before some beginning resolution of the virus was achieved seem ill-advised.

I was surprised at how well psychotherapy, psychoanalysis, and consultation went during this time. I had a previous relationship with everyone I worked with before the pandemic forced us to meet virtually or by phone. I was not working with strangers. I was working with people I knew well, and they knew me well. I could tell my aging brain was influencing my responses, and I felt around the age of eighty would be it for me. The ending was, and still is, quite a loss for me. So much of my identity has been tied to my professional organizations, teaching, and, most importantly, providing psychodynamic forms of treatment.

I well understood Mary's difficulty relinquishing her professional role. But her obsessive work, leading to emotional exhaustion and then anger towards the people she loves, was problematic. I knew my retirement would touch all of this in her.

* * *

During one of our last sessions, she brings up my last day of work.

"So, June 30th is your last day. I've made arrangements with my family physician to prescribe my Lexapro. I have tried tapering off, but I sense that my brain needs it. I have more energy, and I'm less anxious when I take it.

"So, why do you need to retire? You're healthy. You are able to work. It's not fair. I want to see you until one of us dies. Why can't we do that? You have said that you are aware of changes secondary to aging, but I don't see that, except your white hair. Look, this isn't fair. How can you leave me? And NO, I don't want to see somebody else. I just want to keep on seeing you."

"It's painful to say goodbye, for both of us, and being able to love is of immense importance. It isn't easy to accept that there is a time for everything."

"I know we can't be friends. I understand the boundary thing, but I have these loving feelings. That's a good thing, right? I need to keep telling you what I feel, even if I know it's not realistic. Well, I don't want you to retire, get older, or get sick. I want you to stay just as you are. I don't want you to leave me."

"This is connected to so many events in your life."

"Yes, I lost my father to alcohol. I lost my first husband to his PTSD. I lost my brother. I lost my business, and now you're telling me that I'm holding on too tightly to my professional identity? So yes, I don't want to accept your retirement. And you're right; I don't want to give up my professional position. Maybe I can make some changes so I'm not overcommitted, but still, retain a connection to my profession. Maybe it's not that complicated. I could just decide what activities are most rewarding for me and let the other responsibilities go. Saying goodbye to you for the last time will be difficult and sad."

# Chapter Three: KEN

KEN WALKS INTO MY OFFICE and carefully chooses a chair. He is in his late-forties, casually and tastefully dressed, polite, and hesitant. We begin our first session.

"Hi, Dr. Furedy. A friend of my wife recommended you." He pauses, "So here I am in your office, and I don't know what to say."

"Try speaking to what's most on your mind."

"Okay. I'm upset and unhappy and have been this way for years. I just don't know what to say. I get angry so easily and I frequently think about suicide, but I have no plans and I don't want to die. I want to escape the way I feel."

"Are you saying you have experienced these feelings for years and it's much worse now?"

"Yeah, it's much worse. I work in the sales department of a technology firm and I don't like the work. I hate being there. I don't think my sales numbers are adequate and I'm concerned that they are thinking about letting me go. I just have no motivation to do the work. I hate the work. I don't know what's wrong with me.

I don't understand why I have no interest in working. This is not me. I usually muscle through it, but I can't this time. It's a competitive field and my colleagues are highly motivated. I feel defeated."

"Have you thought about the possibility that you might be struggling with depression?"

"I'm not sure that I know what depression is, but I have no energy. I'm not very interested in working on anything at home and I'm kind of hard on my wife and children. The four of them tell me I am so angry and that I lose my temper easily."

"That sounds difficult for all of you. Might there be something else going on that might be affecting you?"

"Well, I do drink quite a bit of whiskey. My wife tells me my mood gets worse after drinking. My father died in his late fifties and he was an alcoholic. He was upset most of the time, wouldn't get involved with the family, and socialized with women he met at bars. He gave my mother barely enough money to take care of our family. Most of his money was spent on alcohol and women. My mother was always upset."

"This must be difficult for you to talk about. Do you wonder if you are an alcoholic like your father and if your anger is being influenced by alcohol? How much drinking do you do on any given day?"

"Oh, it's not too much, maybe half a bottle of whisky. Sometimes I might drink a whole bottle on Saturday and Sunday. Many of my friends drink as much as I do. I don't think it's a serious problem, but it could be contributing to the way I feel."

"Ken, the amount of alcohol you are consuming is excessive. Only an alcoholic can develop the liver enzymes to process such a large amount of alcohol. I think it is highly likely that your use of alcohol is contributing a great deal to your unhappiness. Have you ever considered attending Alcoholics Anonymous? Attending a meeting allows you to listen to the lives of other people who have concluded that alcohol has created serious problems for them. Listening to how ordinary people have struggled with an alcohol addiction can be very useful and help you to not feel so alone with this illness."

"I have considered it, but I've been reluctant to take the steps. I'd feel intense shame if I were an alcoholic like my father. I don't want to be an alcoholic like him."

"There are thousands of individuals who have effectively addressed their addiction to alcohol. If you address your alcohol addiction, your father's destiny does not need to be your destiny."

"Well, I'll consider going to AA meetings. I just don't know how much that's going to help. I have more problems going on besides alcohol."

"Yes, there is more going on. There's so much for us to talk about. Your situation is very complicated. Let's start meeting weekly and we'll take it step by step. It takes considerable courage to start therapy and face such painful issues. I look forward to seeing you next week."

"What! Wait a minute, are you telling me that I must attend AA meetings?"

"It's not for me to instruct or direct you. My role is to comment on what you are saying to me, and try to use my knowledge and understanding to help you, and join you on this journey. Everyone's life is massively complicated, and I can't possibly know what you should do. We will work together to come to some understanding as to why you are so unhappy. I'll see you next week."

The session ends and I feel surprisingly sad and not offended by his outburst. I am worried about Ken. He is in a world of hurt, and for a physician to suggest that someone may be an alcoholic like his father, must have enhanced his emotional pain. My assessment is that meeting in once-a-week psychotherapy will be inadequate to provide the emotional support and understanding he needs, and I will recommend meeting twice a week. In my mind, he is a serious alcoholic, has been for maybe decades, and without my actively addressing this addiction, there will be little chance for him to benefit from psychotherapy. My years of working with alcoholics, while working in multiple hospitals, are informing my understanding and decisions. Alcoholics Anonymous can reduce his shame when he recognizes that other very decent individuals are also struggling with alcohol addiction. My hope is these meetings will provide emotional support, acceptance of his addiction, and solidify the moral core of his being.

* * *

During our second meeting, Ken talks about attending AA meetings.

"I attended some AA meetings and as best as I can determine, listening to other members of the group, I'm an alcoholic. I am addicted to alcohol. Alcohol is causing me to act in ways that are not in anyone's best interest. So far, many of the stories I have heard have similarities to my story. I noticed a number of members have been attending meetings for years. They still have emotional difficulties they are working on, but their lives are going better and they say that they feel and are healthier. I plan on stopping alcohol, but that won't solve most of my problems. The truth is, I feel like shit just about every day. I don't feel like working. I hide out at home watching TV and pornography, and I feel horrible. What type of person am I? I used to be physically active and hardworking. I thought of myself as successful and I don't feel that way about myself anymore."

"Do you think we could say that you are keenly disappointed with yourself and are feeling a great deal of shame?"

"Yes. My wife is doing well. My children are doing extremely well in school. What am I accomplishing? I never liked this job. I'm probably going to be fired."

At this point, I take a careful depression history because I think Ken is probably profoundly depressed. Usually, I will wait a few months to see how withdrawing from alcohol affects the individual. Also, given the frequency of his suicidal ideation and the depth of his despair, I decided to temporarily start a benzodiazepine tranquilizer to help with any withdrawal symptoms.

The next week Ken is calmer but even more depressed. A few weeks later, after most of the alcohol withdrawal symptoms had subsided, I decided to start duloxetine, an antidepressant that increases the central nervous systems serotonin and norepinephrine levels.

A week later, Ken tells me the combination of the benzodiazepine tranquilizer and antidepressant made him feel calmer, and he is sleeping better. He tells me his employer is laying off staff, including him, and that while he feels relieved, he also feels like a failure. He asks both of us why he is not able to motivate himself?

I explain that the alcohol, the depression, and the keen dislike for the company and the products he was selling all came together to paralyze him. I tell him being laid off might help him feel better since he has found no meaning or pleasure in the work he is doing. This might help him return to his old, motivated self and find some clarity of purpose.

Not only was I speaking to what I believed to be true, but I was also remembering the therapist must convey optimism. Ken has just started to lean into the treatment and trust me. How I verbally and nonverbally respond is part and parcel of the therapeutic process. If the patient internalizes the interpersonal process of therapy, this internalization can influence the emotional programs residing in his mind. I felt compassion for him, given how miserable and frightened he was.

As the therapeutic process is internalized, taken into the patient's mind, more adaptive, hopeful structures are created. This is a topic of much discussion and research in my field of study. I tell Ken to achieve his therapeutic goals, he and I must commit considerable time and work to helping him understand himself.

By committing to psychotherapy and medication, the outcome could result in the stabilization of his neurobiology and the development of a non-critical self-exploration and understanding. My curiosity, my optimism, my compassion for his situation, and my attempts to understand in a nonjudgmental manner, if internalized by Ken, may modify his self-criticism, his shame, his feeling of self-disgust, and his anger.

I ask him if other members of his family struggle with depression. He said his father was clearly depressed most of the time, and he feels his mother is unhappy and chronically angry. I think, to myself, that both parents might struggle with a neurobiological proneness towards depression.

* * *

For Ken, the AA Christian orientation is a key blessing since he is, and always has been, deeply religious. Given that God is an entity in his mind, our talking about his relationship with God, and God's expectations for him, has facilitated his progress.

The patient's clarity of religious belief allows the therapist to directly address the patient's relationship with God. It is essential that the therapist sets aside all of his or her beliefs regarding religion, as a way to meld with, and join the suffering mind of the patient to find his way and to discover what is meaningful to him, a core aspect of self-esteem, and dealing with shame and guilt.

I felt the AA meetings were helping Ken to feel closer to God and God's values. I tell Ken the more connected he feels to God, the more he will feel God's blessing and approval. When treating highly religious individuals, I have learned, from the wisdom of colleagues, to respect and accept the relationship with God in the mind of the patient. I did not understand this early in my career.

* * *

Six months have passed and Ken is completely abstinent from alcohol. He attends AA meetings two or three times a week, and we meet twice a week. We have stopped the benzodiazepine tranquilizer since he is no longer in alcohol withdrawal. Ken complains of still feeling sluggish, having no energy or motivation. I decided an increase in his central nervous system norepinephrine and serotonin levels might help. I increased the dose of the duloxetine to increase these levels.

As the months pass, it appears that this medication, along with AA and the psychotherapy, is resulting in him having more energy, less anxiety, less depression, less anger, and less self-destructive impulses. He tells me he is not suicidal. He also continues to benefit from the AA groups, where other attendees are also struggling with depression and their craving for alcohol.

Ken arrives for a session and tells me, "I was finally released from my job, which was a blow to my self-confidence, but also a relief. I wasn't interested in the product and saw no usefulness in it to my customers. I'll work at Costco to help pay the bills until I decide what to do next."

* * *

We have now been working together for one year and he is more stabilized. Our working alliance has been established. He trusts me and I trust him. Together, we are attempting to understand his mind. In the beginning, I did not believe he was emotionally ready to explore his childhood since the depression and withdrawal symptoms were quite intense. I thought he might now be ready. I ask him about his childhood.

Ken was born in Naples, Italy, and is the oldest of five siblings. The family moved from one place to another because of his father's difficulty maintaining employment. He has many cousins with whom he still feels close. He was the leader of his group of friends, who were involved in some mischief, but also did some legitimate work to earn money. He was known as the one in his group who could obtain money, which was a source of childhood pride.

He remembers loving both of his parents, but his father was gone most of the time, and his mother was critical of him for being out with his friends too much. He felt close to the maternal side of his family. His paternal side was more critical and more demanding. Because they lived in a remote area and were not very available, he spent most of his childhood with his maternal extended family in the city.

Although he did not take school too seriously, he did okay. There was one pivotal occasion when an uncle sexually molested him. This was a deep recovery of a repressed memory. He had trouble functioning for several days after remembering this incident. Ken is heterosexual, and the impression I received was that he was raped by an uncle he trusted. This traumatic event added to his difficulty trusting anyone, including himself.

When he was about seven, his nuclear family all immigrated to the United States. His family settled permanently in California's San Fernando Valley. He appeared to adjust to American culture and English and settled into school. Once again, he became a leader of school kids who attempted to make money doing odd jobs and pursuing mischief. His father continued his drinking patterns and was absent most of the time drinking and having sex with other women. When he was a teenager, his parents divorced, and he lived with his mother, brother, and sisters. He told me, "My father was pretty much gone."

The house the family lived in was too small for a family with two teenage boys and two sisters. On his own, he built an extra room, installing the drywall, plumbing, cabinets, and electricity. He enjoyed the building process and started paying attention to the construction of other homes in his neighborhood.

While attending college, he started selling real estate to make money for himself and his family. During this time, he arranged for his family to purchase and move into a larger house. He was able to handle the escrow and other legal aspects of the move. He continued to hang around with his group of friends, many with ties to gangs. His best friend died a violent death while trying to stop two gangs involved in a gang war. After the funeral, he visited the gravesite and promised he would live the rest of his life honoring his friend, who shared the same first name as Ken.

Ken kept his promise to his deceased friend. He finished college and completed graduate school. He met his wife at a party in California. They married and moved to the Puget Sound area, where his wife had family living. They both obtained jobs: she at a local corporation and he in sales. The two of them loved each other, were always committed and faithful. They both were and are deeply religious. I think the moral, trusting, and compassionate teachings of his church helped Ken to organize his thinking and emotions. His clear ability to love, care, and be loyal to his wife and children is an impressive accomplishment, given his father's history. His religious beliefs contributed to defining who he was, but it was much more than religion; this man had an active role in creating himself. Remember, he promised his friend at the gravesite, that he would honor him by being him, representing him. What an amazingly creative solution. I am still impressed.

* * *

With his depression better, his abstinence from alcohol under control, and his deep trust in our work together, we were now able to pursue more intrapsychic emotional conflicts.

Ken felt like a failure professionally. He was a salesman, now working at a reduced level in a warehouse, and felt none of it had meaning other than to make some money. I noticed he would frequently mention houses he drove by, and he was keenly interested in the house I had built and had moved my office to. I did not sense much envy, but more of a keen interest in the architecture, the building process, and the financial processes. I commented on his interest, and he agreed that ever since he had built that room as an addition to his parent's house, he has always been interested in all aspects of building, owning, remodeling, buying, and selling houses. I said, "Is it possible you might be describing your life's work?" He was quiet and slightly nodded in agreement. He needed me to mirror an aspect of himself so he could see and accept this facet of who he *is*.

His wife's job required them to return to Southern California. He joined a real estate development firm with a solid reputation, and started designing, planning, and advertising real estate projects. It was a natural fit, and he soon developed a reputation as a man of considerable knowledge in his field. All of his education, prior experience in sales, and his genuine interest in families finding homes, construction of houses, and architecture all came together. It was enjoyable and meaningful to him to help others find their homes. He had finally found meaning and pride in his work.

His move to California required us to continue his treatment virtually using Zoom. The pandemic had just started, which helped us both accept the necessary reality of virtual communication. Since we had a solid working relationship, the transition from in-person to virtual meetings was fine.

Not long after his move, his emotional conflicts, vulnerable self-esteem, and competition with other colleagues who were more successful than him began to emerge. The money was not enough, although it was substantial. He would overextend himself to his clients as if they were friends and then was angry, secondary to feeling hurt and betrayed by the client who did not act like a grateful friend. The therapy was useful to him to help him put into words what he was feeling and express his impulsive wishes to retaliate against clients not responding as grateful friends.

He was able to use our dialogue to contain his feelings instead of putting them into action. He told me, "It was like they had raped me," an unconscious reference to sexual abuse by his uncle, whom he believed loved him. The amount of money was never enough. He wanted to be the boy who was the leader of the gang, who knew where the money was and could obtain it. Connecting these childhood experiences to his ambitious money thirst was useful to him and helped him to be more realistic. It was more his intense competition that we were looking at, no longer his self-contempt and shame.

* * *

We are now starting the fourth year of his psychotherapy. His depression is stable. He accepts his alcoholism and, with his sobriety, he is now able to help others in AA. In addition, he has regained his love of work.

What about his capacity to love, and his capacity to be self-reflective versus externalizing his painful feelings?

His father dealt with his inner world by becoming intoxicated and disappearing. This ultimately led to his father's early death in his late fifties. His mother kept the family together, and his sisters and brother struggled with their own emotional problems and divorces. His mother, the center of the family, was and is a person who massively externalizes her inner turmoil. When she is upset, the whole family is upset. She tends to blame others, especially Ken, whom I believe has been the object of his mother's displaced anger towards her ex-husband, Ken's father. She demonstrates minimal self-reflection. Ken is always upset when he visits his mother and feels barely able to contain and control his emotions. He finds his mother chaotic and disorganized, and his wish to please her practically always leads to her criticizing him for some misdeed now or in the past.

Ken appears to have internalized this angry, critical maternal object and, at times, treats himself and others in his family in a similar manner as his mother. It appears that his mother resides in the center of his super-ego, available to angrily criticize him and those he loves. Stopping alcohol has helped tremendously, but this necessary depth of self-understanding requires psychodynamic psychotherapy. When we discovered that he was acting like his mother with his own family, he first rejected the concept, and then he accepted the accuracy of it. He felt guilty and ashamed. But he felt he could not control it, especially with his wife.

Because there was so much turmoil in the marriage, his wife Jennifer began requesting to join Ken in therapy. I told Ken that I would need to meet virtually and privately with his wife for a number of visits before we could consider converting to couples psychotherapy. Both the husband and wife agree to this arrangement and I meet individually with Jennifer.

My ability and willingness to consider couples therapy is partly a result of my beginning my professional journey as a family therapist. Few analysts would agree to such an arrangement, viewing it as interfering with the capacity of the analyst to interpret Ken's emotional conflicts and interpret the transference. Usually, I would refer the couple to another therapist. But they had just moved to a different state, the pandemic made all therapy virtual, and my intuitive sense of them was couples therapy most likely would work. Also, and probably the most important factor, was that Ken and Jennifer had decided working with me as a couple would be best for them.

* * *

During my first meeting with Jennifer, she spoke of her husband as being frequently upset and angry. Often, she does not know why he is so upset, but it almost always seemed to be something she had said or done.

She says, "He seems so sensitive, and gets so easily frustrated that it's hard to be around him. Since he stopped drinking and began attending AA and therapy, I don't worry about him as much. I believe he will be okay, but at times, he is impossible to be around. He seems almost always disappointed with me and sometimes with the children. When there are disappointments or frustrations at his work, it's like he dumps it all out at home with little regard for the impact on us, or he withdraws and is sullen."

I think, but do not say, that he is unconsciously recreating his childhood family, acting in ways that are like his mother. Through treatment, he has understood and relinquished much of replicating his father's highly self-destructive behavior. It now sounds like he is, out of awareness, acting through identification, quite a bit like his mother. When he is unhappy, his style of dealing with this is to unconsciously externalize the unhappiness onto his family. He gets them to feel what he is feeling.

I asked Jennifer to tell me about her childhood. She was a fifth-born, first daughter to an immigrant family. Her family came from an influential, wealthy family. Her parents' marriage was arranged, and they moved to the United States to further their education, live safely, and pursue a prosperous life. Her father was a professional man working in the Seattle-Tacoma area. Her mother was intelligent and was always a stay-at-home mother. Jennifer felt loved by both parents and believes her parents wanted her to achieve in a manner similar to her siblings.

Jennifer did well in school, attended a university, worked in a similar field as her father, and married Ken in her early twenties. When her children were young teenagers, she returned to work in her discipline. She has been very successful at work and has recently been advanced to an administrative position involving legal and financial decisions. Unlike her husband, who dislikes having a boss he must report to, she manages these relationships well. Her interpersonal skills are well developed.

When she was latency age (ages seven to twelve), her father started an affair with a neighbor. She remembers the neighborhood kids knowing about the affair, along with her family, extended family, and friends. Eventually, her parents divorced, but her father continued financially supporting her mother and his children's education. She remains emotionally close to both of her parents. It was difficult for her to move to California because of her work. She wanted to stay close to her family of origin.

* * *

We start couples therapy, which replaces all individual work. Both Ken and Jennifer wish to continue using couples therapy. They both feel they are better able to attend to emotional problems using this format. This was a new experience for me. I have, many times, had the spouse join the treatment, but treatment always reverted to individual psychotherapy with the spouse who originally sought treatment. However, this couple expressed their individual assessment that they could gain more from working together as a couple than individually. I have learned to accept that the work is conjoint; the work is intersubjective, and the working alliance is never about my possessing superior knowledge. It's an interpersonal type of work, where understanding emerges and hopefully is accepted by, in this case, all three members of the therapeutic team.

Their first session as a couple is a portent of all future sessions. Ken always leaves the topic to be discussed to his wife, Jennifer. For example, she started one session by describing a family outing.

"You were driving with all five of us in the car. You became upset that the car in front of you was going too slowly, so you blasted your horn, sped around him, and then gave him the finger. I was scared and so were our children."

Ken states, "We had reservations, and we were going to be late. You made the arrangements and there wasn't enough time. If we were late, once again, I would look foolish, and I would be upset. What did you expect me to do?"

Jennifer responds to Ken with a recommendation. "I have been reading this book on mindfulness, and if you would only read this book and learn how to calm yourself."

* * *

I thought and felt that Ken was definitely an emotional handful, and Jennifer lectures him as if he were an employee at work having problems. She is providing instruction, and believes she knows the correct way for her husband to handle himself. I once mentioned that I had a friend struggling with intense shame, having her husband in mind. She recommended a book to me on shame she had read in one of her corporate improvement classes.

After watching these types of interactions for many sessions, I concluded that Ken was unconsciously looking for approval and emotional support from his capable wife. Instead of what he longed for, he received lectures, information, directions, and advice. I never heard comments from Jennifer such as, "You felt you would embarrass the entire family if you were late." Or, "Oh, you discovered your colleague made more sales than you did, so you felt defeated. The money you make is great. We don't need anymore." The emotional content is seldom addressed, as was the case in her childhood family. In her family of origin, no one ever talked about how her father's affair had massively impacted the family.

Part of the difficulty this couple was having was cultural. They came from two very different cultures. One culture highly valued the expression of emotions, while the other culture highly valued the controlled, rational, disciplined approach. I may be overemphasizing the impact of the cultural differences, but I think I am not exaggerating the emotional patterns that these two kind-hearted individuals grew up in.

Multiple times I said, "Jennifer, you are attempting to give your husband instructions on how you believe he should solve this particular problem. Without being aware of it, you don't focus and acknowledge what he is experiencing, what he is feeling." I would often say to Ken, "You learned to spew your feelings out. You are trying to get your wife to feel what you are feeling. You are not aware that you are doing this, but you are. You learned this from your family, just like Jennifer learned from her family, to speak only to logic and solutions, not emotions."

Jennifer is very kind, and the more she could tune into the emotions of her husband and put into words what he was feeling, such as "You are frustrated, feel like you don't measure up to your colleagues, your feelings are hurt, and you didn't feel loved," the less Ken spewed out and externalized his feelings.

As Ken began making more statements about himself rather than others, he increased his capacity to conceptualize his feelings and put them into words. This led him to modify his old pattern of action-prone behavior to escape from his intolerable feelings.

Jennifer also became curious about her feelings and became able to talk about her sadness and concern regarding many aspects of her family. The responsibilities of her work increased, secondary to her success at work, and at times, she would feel overwhelmed and unsure of herself. She used the therapy and was able to use her husband as someone who could calm her. He became a source of potential comfort, not always an emotional tornado.

* * *

After about two years of couples therapy, we finished our work. Vestiges of the old patterns remained, but they both had a better understanding and combined capacity to work together. She was now more comfortable with emotionally tuning in, and he was now more comfortable identifying what he might be feeling, and expecting that his wife would listen and understand, most of the time. They developed considerable empathic listening skills for each other and themselves.

# Chapter Four: TED

TED AND HIS WIFE Jane, both in their mid-to-late thirties, arrive for their first appointment. Jane is attractive, animated, and charming. She is also very angry with her husband. She complains he does no cooking, house cleaning, or yard work. She says he spends too much time playing and watching sports with their children. She uses the session to vent her frustrations about her husband. This couple had been separated for several months and was coming to see me as part of their attempt to save their marriage. She is adamant that she does not need couples therapy. Jane is bringing her husband for treatment.

Ted speaks rapidly, uses psychological terms, quotes his previous psychiatrist, and is clearly very anxious.

I leave the first session feeling confused and call his previous psychiatrist, who had moved to Minnesota and was no longer available to Ted, except for occasional phone contact. Dr. Alan tells me he did not believe continuing his therapy by phone was in Ted's best interest. He had started seeing Ted when he was a child in middle school and was having panic attacks, which led to school refusal. Between Ativan, a minor benzodiazepine tranquilizer, and weekly psychotherapy, Ted returned to school, and later graduated from college. Ted is presently working in the profession in which he received his degree. As I think about my next meeting with this couple, I continue to feel quite perplexed.

Ted and Jane return for their second session and the dialogue feels like a repetition of the first meeting. Jane continues with her long list of complaints about what Ted does not do, and Ted speaks in sentences that are not connected to the conversation. This time I feel his anxiety, and I can again feel Jane's intense anger. I suggest that maybe my meeting twice a week with Ted might be the best way to proceed. My thinking is, given how fractured their relationship is, I doubt I could form a working alliance with them as a couple.

Jane enthusiastically said, "Yes! I have my own therapist. My husband needs treatment."

* * *

Ted arrives for the third session and is a bit more relaxed meeting with me alone. He fills the session with a detailed history of his childhood and how his psychiatrist, Dr. Alan, had helped him. I feel like he is telling me a story, and less like he is telling me his story.

He tells me his parents divorced when he was about ten. His father lost his job, most likely because he was always drinking alcohol and could not function very well. Ted's use of alcohol is infrequent and never excessive. He does not have any history of drug abuse. Instead of identifying with this aspect of his father, as a teenager, he consciously decided he would not become an alcoholic, like his father.

During the session, I decided to attempt exploring his understanding of his father's dysfunction, knowing he had previously been in psychotherapy.

"Your doctor prescribed Ativan, which is used for anxiety. Do you think it's possible that your father also struggled with extreme anxiety? Do you think he might have been trying to self-medicate with alcohol?"

Ted responds, "I don't know. I never thought about it in that way, maybe so."

I recommended changing the Ativan to a longer-acting benzodiazepine to deal with his anxiety. I tell him, "If you take this new medication only at night, once you have mastered a situation, you will be less likely to attribute your success to the immediate availability of the Ativan." He agrees to this change. He has been on benzodiazepines for at least fifteen years, and dealing with benzodiazepine withdrawal would be very difficult for any patient, and would be the last thing he needed at this time.

* * *

We start meeting twice a week, combined with 2 mg of clonazepam, a long-acting benzodiazepine, which he takes at night. As his anxiety improved and knowing I was available to him, he began calming down and trusting me. I was now better able to understand him. He explained to me that he had been trying to tell me everything he had learned in his work with Dr. Alan. He acknowledged it might have been difficult for me to follow his thinking.

I now understood that he was feeling panicked during our first few meetings. He also believed he needed to perform and demonstrate all that he had learned during his treatment with Dr. Alan. I was relieved. He was not psychotic, and I was dealing with an anxiety disorder with the defensive activity of dissociation associated with an as-if form of performing. He was acting as if he understood himself.

Ted has a severe anxiety disorder with attempts to perform. This has been his adaptation since childhood and has probably resulted in others experiencing him as if he is not speaking coherently. He is performing and can be disconnected from his emotions and the content of his sentences. As a result, others, including myself, might feel immense confusion when trying to understand him. He has an elaborate, as-if defensive character structure. When performing, he dissociates and has little connections to his emotions and, at times, his thinking. This was my tentative understanding of why I could not follow his words during our first two meetings. His dissociated way of performing, starting in childhood, led to his difficulty being and knowing himself. He tended to look to others for direction and approval and affirmation of who he was. He performed in a manner compatible with what he believed others wanted. This ultimately rendered him passive, compliant, and anxious.

We work well together, and I like him. He is a kind, honest man with much integrity. He is also passive, dependent, and boy-like. He relates to his wife as if she were a mother. As a child and adolescent, he experienced his mother as chronically angry with his father. His mother was very demanding of Ted and expected him to excel in academics and sports. For his mother, Ted was what is referred to as a narcissistic object. He was a source of social pride for her. His considerable success in sports led to her gaining a great amount of positive attention. She was delighted with the attention and praise she received from other parents: "Oh, you are Ted's mother. He's the star of the team."

As his math and science classes became more demanding, obtaining straight A's was not as easy. He became panicked, knowing his mother would be disappointed if his performance was not outstanding. He unconsciously expected he would be rejected, as his father had been, for not measuring up to her expectations.

* * *

Six months into Ted's treatment, he decided to leave his administrative position because his anxiety was so intense when he was required to make decisions he alone could make. I connected his performance anxiety to his father's rejection for not measuring up to his mother's expectations. I began to understand that pleasing the maternal object in his mind was how he sought direction. Please mother, or some current representation of the mother, and you will be safe.

He chose another more technical job and continued to be very anxious and unsure of himself.

His wife's anger did not subside. He discovered she was having multiple affairs and spending excessive amounts of money. She angrily criticized him daily. I interpreted to him that he was very psychologically dependent on his wife like he was with his mother.

Ted had concluded as a young adolescent that meeting his mother's expectations would prevent him from being rejected and devalued like his father. All of this was understood through the mind and eyes of a young teenager and had unconsciously continued into adulthood. His young adolescent understanding was being superimposed on his dissolving marriage and his wife's ongoing anger. Through his adolescent mind, he thought pleasing and performing for his wife-mother would be the correct path. His wife, considering whom she chose for her second husband, was looking for a man who was aggressive and took charge, not a man obsequiously trying to please her.

I understood that my job required me to be emotionally present, tuned into his emotional experience with himself, put into words and concepts, his experience of himself, and avoid giving advice. He did not need a parent-therapist whose expectations were to be met. He continuously tried to read me verbally and nonverbally, looking for clues for directions and approval. His actual father was too damaged and viewed as inferior to help Ted psychologically separate from his mother and become his own person. Part of the function of fathering is to help the child safely attach to the father to facilitate the needed process of psychological individuation. Ted had definitely not accomplished individuation, so I knew my job was to provide emotional mirroring to help him see and experience himself.

Eventually, Jane filed for divorce after spending considerable amounts of money buying expensive items, including a luxury car. She knew Ted would be legally responsible for most of the debt. The divorce proceeded.

At first, he allowed his wife to choose his lawyer, and then complained that his lawyer appeared to only agree with his wife. It was more like she was not his attorney, but his wife's attorney. I interpreted, "You are more comfortable doing what you are told, like with your mother, instead of obtaining a lawyer whom you experience as legally representing you." He agreed. He found another lawyer, a man who he felt understood and who was actively representing him. The divorce proceeded and the family court granted joint custody of the three children.

Ted was now single, financially, just okay, and had an equal amount of time with his children. The start-up company he worked for financially dissolved, and he found another job in his field. To his surprise, he felt socially more at ease in his new job and was aware he occasionally advised some of his younger colleagues. While he felt the same anxiety, it was less intense, and it did not stop him from proceeding in most areas of life.

I would say to him, "There is considerable pleasure and fun being you, and believing in yourself." He knew that I believed in his abilities. I suspect this was communicated at a non-verbal level since I was very careful not to be particularly supportive or encouraging. He did feel that his father believed in him, but his father was drunk much of the time and died when he was in college. Ted replicated some aspects of his father. His father was kind, passive, and a failure in everybody's eyes, including Ted's. The reality of his impaired and mostly absent father made it nearly impossible for Ted to soundly identify with his father and psychologically separate from his mother. He developed a style of performing for his mother and maternal aunt, regardless of what he thought or felt.

Out of Ted's psychological necessity, I became, within the paternal transference, the father he could comfortably identify with. Another way to conceptualize this is I became a paternal developmental object that facilitated individuation, a function that his impaired father could not provide. In his transference to me, at an unconscious level, he experienced me as the competent missing father that he could be with. I understood the transference but did not interpret it at this time, since he was dealing with so much in his present personal life, and he was benefiting from the paternal transference to me, as a competent father.

* * *

In defiance of the family court agreement, his ex-wife moved to a different state and took his two younger children. He now only had Zoom to meet regularly with his two children, while his firstborn was starting college. He missed them terribly and considered pursuing legal action. He met with his lawyer and the two of them decided trying to gain full custody of his children would probably not be successful. The state his ex-wife moved to would never remove children from a mother who was a registered nurse and had no legal violations. He knew he had been manipulated, but felt pride in actively choosing his lawyer and actively engaging in these important decisions for his children and his relationship with them.

The company he now worked for merged with another company. To keep his position in the newly merged company, he was required to move to another state. Not wanting to move, he quickly applied to another company and was accepted for a job that required considerable technical expertise and administrative responsibilities. To Ted's surprise, his leadership skills were growing. He developed and led five technical groups. He did not feel anxious, and he could tell that both his male and female colleagues respected and trusted him. He felt little anxiety. He believed in himself, his abilities, and his judgment.

In my mind, after about two years of twice-a-week psychodynamic psychotherapy, he had internalized the psychotherapeutic process, which involves some identification with his therapist. The reflective aspect of the work allowed Ted to emotionally see himself. He no longer needed to be a performing "son" for me, as the transference mother.

So, what about his sex life? He had been a virgin before he married, and he wanted to have some adventures after his divorce. His first move in this area was to join a Bible study group where his tendency to perform, be dependent and seek direction from older women led him to accept the moral directive of an older female group leader. The message was clear: no sexual activity should occur until marriage. He had received the same lecture from his mother and aunt, who both equated premarital sex with sexual promiscuity.

The message interfered markedly with feeling comfortable dating. I asked him if he believed in what the Bible study group leader had told him. He said he was unsure, but he remembered many of his teenage friends being sexually active, and their parents did not seem upset about it. After his parents' divorce, his father had a number of female friends. Maybe he did not agree that being sexually active was sinful, as the Bible study leader implied. He still struggled with his guilt about his sexual wishes and his attraction to women. On his own, he said, "Maybe, once again, I am behaving like a good boy, and not staying with what I want and believe."

Ted was anxious about interacting with women and did not come across as genuine. He reverted to his acting as-if role. This was not successful because the women could intuitively sense that he was not genuine.

He felt guilty and ashamed of his sexual impulses towards available women. The more experience he gained, the more chances he took, the more his anxiety dissipated, and the more we analyzed his beliefs, guilt, and shame regarding his sexual interest in women. He became more self-confident with his sexual ability and sexual attractiveness. In his discussions with me, it was hard for him to admit he was not looking for a wife. He knew I was married, and believed I expected him to marry, but he wanted to be his own man, not my compliant son.

Ted wanted sexual friendships and adventure. He wanted to experience what he had missed as a teenager and young adult. He dated a number of women, tried living with one, but did not feel ready to make a lifetime commitment. His anxiety about interacting with women became greatly diminished. He enjoyed sports, hiking, dating, and sex. His anxiety at work also faded, and he gravitated to leadership roles, more evidence of his emotional maturation.

* * *

The medical insurance available with his new employer did not cover ongoing psychotherapy. After using the twenty visits available, he concluded he was ready to stop therapy because of how well he was doing. He had emotionally dissociated from his feelings about the reality of my announced retirement in a number of months. He was unconsciously attempting to use his familiar dissociative mechanisms: "I'm fine, and I'm not upset or have strong feelings about your retirement."

This did not work, and he regressed, flooded with fear and sadness. He had been disconnected from his feelings. He emotionally experienced and then understood that he was not accepting that I would no longer be available. He regressed and felt intense sadness, fear, and loneliness. He was overwhelmed by the intensity of his complicated emotional response to my no longer being available. As he regressed and felt more terrified, he went back to speaking in a dissociative, performing manner. Luckily, we recognized what was occurring. He had been denying the emotional impact of my retirement on him, even though he had known about it for two years.

He felt the terror of separation. He recognized it, and then I recognized it, and we were both able to share the experience of the loss and sadness of knowing we would be ending our meetings soon. Within a week, he was back on track. He was forced to face and work through the grief of losing his father-therapist. Ultimately, this temporary intense regression was therapeutic progress. He was able to feel the emotional pain of ending, put his feelings into words, experience and endure the feelings, and eventually share this experience with me. This was progress, although very painful.

Ted's emotional regression led to his realization that as long as he had me, he was not as much in need of a psychologically intimate relationship with someone else. While dating, he kept women at a distance, not completely trusting them. We agreed finding a female psychotherapist for him to work with after our sessions ended would be in his best interest.

* * *

After working together for about five years, there was progress in all areas: better self-confidence, self-understanding, and experience of self. He seldom dissociated or went into performance mode. His capacity to accept and manage responsibility had markedly improved. He better managed his finances and explored sports and activities that he enjoyed. He had more loving connections to members of his family, especially his siblings, and continued to have a loving relationship with his children.

The intense psychodynamic psychotherapy resulted in remarkable changes. He moved from the position of phobic avoidance, dependent relationships, not trusting himself, and avoiding responsibility to accepting leadership roles in his profession, thinking on his own about important issues, like decisions regarding his children, managing his finances, forming friendships with other physically active men, and exploring different possible relationships with women. He made the decision to apply for an advanced position with his employer, which would result in more responsibility, a higher income, and better medical insurance.

He knows he will need to continue working on his keen distrust of women, and his pattern of keeping them at an emotional distance. He and I both agreed that working with an experienced female psychodynamic therapist would better facilitate working through his distrust and fear of loving a woman.

Life is an ongoing process, and no psychotherapy or psychoanalysis will resolve all issues. The human mind is too complicated to ever reach completion.

# Chapter Five: SHELLY

SHELLY, A YOUNG WOMAN in her early twenties, walks into my office for her first appointment. She drops her backpack, full of books, on the floor with a loud thump. She sits on the couch with her arms folded in front of her and looks at me with some defiance.

"Okay, so you're the psychiatrist the ER doctor spoke so highly of. She said you are the best. So, are you?" She quietly pauses. "A friend of my family recommended you, too." She pauses again, and, with an air of boredom, says, "What should I talk about?"

I ask, "Are you in emotional pain?"

"Hell no, that's what the drugs are for. I spent last week with my best friend and we were high on meth all week. You probably disapprove. When I go to raves, I use Ecstasy. I dance, meet guys, and have a great time. You probably don't approve of me using a few joints of marijuana every day, but I feel calm and creative. Besides, I'm able to do my studying. My grades are slipping some. You'll probably blame it on marijuana. If I feel down, I know what to do. I have my drugs. Why would you think your medical drugs are any better than my drugs? Hmm. You're awfully quiet. What do you think?"

"I don't know you yet. I'm reluctant to say much since I don't understand what is occurring in your life and in your mind."

"Come on, it's not that complicated. I'm attending my classes and majoring in an area that interests me. I'm probably brilliant! That's what my mother and my teachers and professors have said to me. I score high on IQ tests, but I'm not doing as well in college as I expected. I came here because my family said I needed help. So, what do you have to say about that?"

I am feeling amused by this young woman as she continues to challenge me. "You want me to give you my opinion when I really don't know you?"

"Sure, tell me what you think, Doc."

"Okay, I'll risk it. You have said I probably disapprove and blame your slipping grades on your drug use. In my world, we call that projecting. I think you might, out of your awareness, be placing your thoughts and concerns on me. The appeal might be that you could then be in an argument with me and win the argument. This might be more appealing to you than the difficulties of dealing with uncertainty."

"So, you think I'd rather argue with you than face my problems?"

"Maybe."

"Hmm, I'll think about that. I think our time is up." Shelly abruptly ends the session as another attempt to challenge me and take control of our dialogue.

Taking control is most likely what she does in most of her relationships. She is correct that she is bright. I wonder if she unconsciously lives with the terror that she could be damaging her brain and, consequently, harming what she believes to be the most valued aspect of herself, her intelligence. At this point, I have no idea if we will be able to form a working alliance.

* * *

During the next four appointments, Shelly does not change her dialogue or positions much. She does agree to meet once a week. I do what I can to not allow my alarm regarding her drug abuse to lead to a paternalistic response from me. I know that individuals with this amount of excessive drug use have their best chance of recovery when the decision belongs to them when it is their conclusion, but I am worried.

In our next session, she says, “We have been meeting for a month and my mother thinks I should admit myself into a rehab program. Do you know of any good programs?”

I answered her question and referenced a local program with a good reputation. She decides to give this program a try but wants to continue to talk to me by phone while in the program. I agree. I am able to see that she is beginning to trust me. I also feel relieved. Her family was actively confronting her drug abuse, which left room for me to maintain an interpretive position. I was not telling her what to do. I was listening, being available as she came to her own decisions.

She spends one month in the inpatient unit, joins an aftercare group, and stops all drugs except for marijuana. She says to me, “How could a small bowl of marijuana possibly do harm? Just one bowl in the evening. What harm could that do? It’s so minor.”

I respond, “In comparison to the total amount of drugs you were using, it seems small to you. What do the members of your group say?”

“They say they understand that I’m frightened of full recovery since I don’t know what life without drugs will be like for me.”

“And your thoughts?”

“Okay. I know I’m hanging onto Mary Jane, but what will I do with all these intense feelings I'm having?"

"It might help you to understand that a large part of your drug use has been to not feel or experience the emotional aspect of yourself. You are now feeling overwhelmed by the intensity of what you're experiencing. You have few words and little understanding of all of this."

I know she is going through withdrawal, and is flooded with feelings and memories she can feel, but has no idea of the content. I make the decision to recommend psychoanalysis. She is in a crisis and will benefit from the psychological holding of meeting four times per week. She is also intelligent and surprisingly psychologically minded. She is developing the capacity to trust me and is forming a working alliance with me. These are qualities that allow a person to be able to benefit from psychoanalysis. She is in crisis and needs intense treatment to survive and benefit from this crisis.

I say to her, "I'm thinking that maybe we should consider meeting four times per week to provide a place, a relationship, where you can bring these intense, overwhelming feelings."

"Okay, I might as well. My life has been turning to shit. I've had to drop most of my classes because I can't think, remember, or do just about anything. My group members say it will pass, but I don't know."

The next few months are primarily about the storm of withdrawal from drugs, with some memories of her past starting to percolate into her conscious mind.

* * *

Over the next year, her story unfolds. A story she had repressed, and the core members of her family, her mother, in particular, had no idea of.

Her parents divorced when she was about seven. Joint custody was agreed to, and there were times when she might spend a week or two with her father. Her father was a drinking alcoholic and a drug user. When she was alone with him, he was always high. At times, her father could not pay for his drugs. Then a repressed memory stormed forward.

She tells me, "There was this one dealer who liked me. My father paid for his drugs by letting this guy have sex with me. He had a gun and sometimes he would stick the gun in my vagina and then tell me to taste the gun. Then he would stick the gun in my bottom and tell me to taste it. He would say, one is sweet, the other tastes bad. Oh my God, my father let this happen to me. Oh my God."

She needed many months to process remembering these traumatic events and experiencing the horrible mixture of overwhelming feelings of her father betraying her and using her for financial gain. The memories, the feelings, the betrayal, the rape were remembered and were available for understanding. Some of the bodily sensations connected to inchoate experiences were felt but not easily translatable into words. The emergence of all these sensations was remembered and consequently became available to the conscious part of her mind/brain so that we could understand in-depth her present-day experiences.

Her father also married another drug user, and Shelly remembers that her stepmother would tell Shelly how to act so that her stepmother could obtain opiates from the ER doctors. (Munchausen syndrome by proxy). She also remembered that dinner was seldom prepared in the evening. Her stepmother was irresponsible, mean, and nasty towards her. Her father and her stepmother divorced about the time Shelly went off to college.

After remembering these events, and realizing her father never paid for any of her education, only her mother and stepfather did, Shelly decided she would "divorce" her father by having no future contact with him. She did this, even though he tried a number of times to make contact with her. When she was able to remember her horrible childhood abuse, lack of parental protection, and his selling her sexually when she was a child, she concluded he had no right to claim that he was her father. She turned over her affection toward her stepfather, who was a good man and cared about her. She also was able to take the risk and feel love toward me.

After three years of psychoanalysis, she was drug-free, graduated from college, and was working in her field. She also chose a boyfriend quite different from the men she used to date. He was not dramatic. He was responsible, loving, hardworking, and very much in love with her.

* * *

During her treatment, I had been attending a study group of psychoanalysts practicing in different cities in the United States and decided to present one of Shelly's sessions to them. In this session, the only thing she talked about was how deeply she loved me, and that she would take a bullet to protect me. She went on and on with how wonderful I was, and again stated she would die to protect me.

The analysts from my study group were not impressed. Why was I not interpreting the transference? Why was I not addressing unconscious conflict, or exploring the meaning of her insistence on love? I told them they did not understand, that this was the emergence of an unconscious childhood longing that she needed to experience to be able to resume her emotional development, which was stunted following the horrible childhood abuse. It was essential that I accept and not disturb her capacity to feel and express love, and not interpret as transference her emotional experience. For Shelly, believing in me and loving me was central to her finding herself, loving herself, being proud of herself, and knowing that she was lovable.

So many individuals with serious drug addictions are never able to obtain this loving state and, consequently, cannot love others, their life, or themselves. It was essential that I not make attempts to be psychoanalytically sophisticated. Instead, I needed to understand how precious and life-sustaining this experience and the telling of this experience was for her. I think, after listening further, the psychoanalysts from my study group finally understood.

Shelly's experience was that of a child adoring and wanting to adore her analyst-father. And, maybe, more importantly, I was what is referred to as a developmental object for her: a therapist being available to facilitate psychological development that had not occurred because she did not have the needed father who should have protected her; but instead, subjected her to massive childhood sexual terrifying trauma.

* * *

Shelly's mother had flaws and anxiety and deeply loved her daughter. She tried to protect her and was horrified when she heard of some of the abuse her daughter experienced under the care of her father and stepmother. Fortunately, her mother's second husband was a kind, loving, steady, intelligent man who loved her mother and her daughter, Shelly.

Several years after Shelly finished her treatment, I was invited and attended her wedding. About three years later, she called and set up a time to bring her one-year-old child to my office. She had left her childhood blanket at my office and was ready to retrieve it. She was doing well and had a loving relationship with her husband and child. I agreed to both of these meetings, post-analysis, since I believe that retaining an image of her analyst as loving, interested, and taking pleasure in her doing well should never, ever be damaged, if humanly possible.

How could an individual recover from such horrific child abuse? Is it innate strength, a loving mother, a present and kind stepfather, a willingness to go through drug recovery, and spend four years in psychoanalysis? Does this explain it all? Is there more to understand? Certainly, these factors are of immense importance, and there is always more to understand. For now, let's thank the universe for providing and helping her find treatments that still have mysteries, but saved the life of a wonderful person.

# Chapter Six: DEBORAH

DEBORAH IS A WOMAN in her mid-thirties who moved to the Seattle area after being laid off by her employer in Boston. During our first meetings, she reveals little information that conveys her understanding as to why she was laid off, other than that she feels like a failure. As far as I can assess, her new job is an advancement, indicating that her new employer views her as experienced and talented, something she does not see in herself. I experience her as a profoundly nice, friendly, and animated woman. She is the type of person most people are drawn to, like, and trust. I also notice that her voice seems too young for a woman of her age. She has a little girl's voice.

She tells me that she had always struggled with anxiety and self-doubt. She had previous psychotherapy from a psychiatrist and is taking sertraline (Zoloft), a selective serotonin reuptake inhibitor (SSRI) antidepressant, which she has concluded helps her to feel less anxious, less depressed, and less discouraged. She says she has a sugar addiction, and if left to her own wishes, she would probably eat only sweets. She is a very slender woman, which is not the usual presentation a clinician finds with a sugar addiction. She says her appearance is very important to her and she would never allow herself to become overweight.

Since moving to the area almost one year ago, she has created no friendships, and she has no boyfriend. She only goes to work and attends a workout class at a local gym. She feels lonely, alone, not attractive, and at a loss for what to do. She wanted to be in treatment with a woman. She met with a female psychoanalyst in Seattle but concluded she was too far from her work and then was referred to me.

She talks freely during our first meeting and has some capacity for self-reflection, probably a result of her previous therapy in Boston.

I comment, "You feel anxious about your ability to handle your new job. You are lonely and tend to isolate yourself and hide out in your condo. Is this correct?"

"Yes, that is correct. I have been a loner most of my life. I've only had one long-term boyfriend when I was in college. He later decided to marry a woman in the same field as him. I doubt that I loved him."

The session is about to end and I say, "We will need to stop today. It does seem as if you are almost frozen and terrified of continuing with your life outside of work. We will need ample time to work on these long-standing emotional difficulties. I recommend we meet twice a week."

She nods in agreement and says, "I will need the appointment times to be later in the day because I cannot miss work."

Before our next meeting, I wonder why she is so anxious, so isolated, so avoidant, and so unsure of herself? She is highly educated and has a graduate degree from an outstanding university. She is smart, attractive, likeable, and appears kind. What is going on in her mind? How did this happen?

For the first few months, she primarily talks about her relationships at work. She excessively worries about her boss and co-workers not liking her or approving of her work. She fills most of her sessions with details about her sophisticated and important work, and her constant worry about what management thinks about her work. I think, to myself, this is obsessional thinking, partly driven by anxiety.

I remind myself that in the beginning, her being able to trust me and work with me, through my careful, empathic listening, is more important than an attempt to uncover etiology. I make statements like, "You are preoccupied with the possibility of disapproval. It's as if disapproval places you in actual danger. You attempt to ward off disapproval by being extra nice. You may be conveying, in your manner of speaking, 'Please don't hurt me'!"

Her response to this intervention was to return to the details of her previous job where she and other colleagues were laid off. "My colleagues did not measure up to expectations, and neither did I." She also comments that she remembers being worried about not measuring up to expectations ever since elementary school.

I think to myself this might be an opportunity to start our exploration of her mind. "Do you remember what grade you were in when this type of worry started?"

"I don't know. It seems like always, but let me think... It probably started in third grade. My teacher was nice, but I became very worried that my work wasn't good enough, and that my classmates didn't like me."

"Third grade? You were probably eight years old? Was there anything else of importance occurring in your life?"

"My little brother was about three years old. He was born with a damaged left ear. My father didn't like him. He saw him as damaged goods and would say stuff like that out loud. He drank a lot and when he was drunk, in particular, he would get very angry.

He'd then yell and complain about having to take care of my brother. At times, he would hit my mother. I was terrified. Once he was so angry that he fired a gun towards my mother and missed her head by inches. She eventually became fed up with him and divorced him.

"I was his favorite. I was his little girl, and I adored him. He was the CEO of a large company in Los Angeles. He was smart, charming, and wealthy. He came from a wealthy family and his mother adored him. I adored him and he adored me until it all went to hell."

I say nothing and continue to listen.

"I became terrified of him and did not want to be around him. The family court judge awarded him visitation, but neither my little brother nor I wanted to be alone with him. If we went to dinner with him, he always got drunk and angry with the waiters. We were terrified. We did everything to avoid being with him, especially alone with him. He would drive his car to our school, park on the street in front of the school, and wait for us after school. He was in violation of a court order, and my mother's lawyer threatened him with legal action if he did not stop. He was stalking us. It was scary and creepy. Even now he will try to follow me on social media, even though I blocked him."

* * *

The next few months of her psychotherapy are filled with these traumatic memories. She reviews in great detail her childhood events, the fear, and her little brother who she feels she must protect.

Her mother, a highly successful physician, is solid, loving, and filled with daily advice, most of which appear to have been realistic and caring. Her family then consisted of three: her mother, brother, and herself. This trio was organized around "mother knows best." Luckily, her mother had good judgment and advice, but it is hard for a child to develop self-confidence and individuation with a frightening, potentially dangerous father. Following her mother's instructions and advice is the safest route. Being a good girl, looking for and following her mother's instructions to avoid danger, does describe the style of how she presents herself in her professional work.

When Deborah was about eleven, her mother remarried a loving, kind, and scholarly man. Deborah psychologically adopted her stepfather as her father and did everything she could to erase all awareness of her biological father, and to never have any contact with him. She and her brother have maintained this no-contact position to this day. They are aware that he has left his employment, has inherited considerable wealth and is now living his life pursuing creative endeavors. Much to my surprise, becoming somebody, like her father, who achieves recognition and fortune, became her unconscious expectation for herself, standards by which she measures her worth. Consciously, she rejects him. Unconsciously, she identifies with his accomplishments and wealth and these become her goals. Again, this is all out of her awareness.

* * *

During the first two years of treatment, I would carefully connect present-day worries and anxiety to her childhood terror. I connected her fear of attack from her bosses to her childhood fear of her father; her self-doubt to always believing that her mother is smarter and knows best; her tendency toward hiding and avoidance of her hiding and avoiding her father when he proved himself to be dangerous; her little girl's voice as an attempt to convey that she needs protection and should not be attacked or punished. She actively worked with me to create this understanding. She experienced and came to understand that our looking closely at her was not to criticize, attack, or find fault, but to understand.

After a few years of therapy, she became more self-confident and was promoted at work, leading to a substantial increase in her income. She made friends at work and started to date. She enjoyed dating, and tended to choose men who were not interested in a commitment, but more interested in sex and fun, which she said was okay with her since she had missed out on dating. Still, she tended to feel unwanted at the end of these relationships, even though she knew that she did not want a long-term commitment from any of these men. It was like there was only one explanation for a relationship to end, and that was rejection, leading her to find proof that she was not wanted.

I sometimes interpreted that even though she knew she was not responsible for her parents' divorce, she probably felt, as with her relationships, somehow responsible for the ending and, ultimately, the loss of a father she had adored. She was intrigued by this idea and began productively exploring her relationships with men, her tendency to hide, to avoid, and now to feel rejected.

At the same time, a submerged symptom became apparent. She was chronically dissatisfied with her work, her accomplishments, and felt not appreciated. Also, her work was not particularly meaningful to her. She was in an important position in a technical department, but she was dissatisfied. She felt no one valued her because she did not have the proper credentials, so she sought out positions in other sectors of the company, sectors that had more of an international focus.

She changed jobs, found considerable recognition, attended high-level prestigious conventions, and still remained dissatisfied. She decided her home was not fancy enough and her salary was too low, even though it placed her in the upper one percent of income earners. Was she depressed? I raised the dose of her medication with no benefit and returned her to her usual maintenance dose after two months. I concluded that this was not a biological depression, but more about how she was processing her experiences at work and her accomplishments. She was never satisfied with herself. I interpreted that she probably projected her dissatisfaction with herself onto others and consequently experienced them as dissatisfied with her.

We began exploring her dissatisfaction.

I comment, "You make a great deal of money. Your retirement plan has a few million. You are doing the work you said you always wanted to do, but you are dissatisfied. How are we to understand this?"

"It's true you don't understand. Look, some of the work I do involves sales. Well, not exactly sales. It involves creating programs so people in this country and others can learn how to use our products. I hate the emphasis on the profit gained by promoting the company's products. I didn't go into this field to be selling products. I did it to help the less advantaged. You say I have enough money, but some of my colleagues live in more beautiful houses than mine, in better locations, and are multimillionaires. I only have a few million. My boss doesn't like or appreciate me, and I've started avoiding going into the office. I don't want to attend her meetings. She doesn't like me."

"Didn't you tell me that your father inherited considerable wealth, and you resented not being included? Do you think it's possible that you are responding to your boss with envy of her wealth and anger like you felt toward your father?"

"Not everything comes from my past. Maybe I just dislike this particular woman. And it IS unfair that she has so much more than I do. Maybe this is just reality and has nothing to do with my father."

"It is something for us both to think about."

She decides it is time to leave her job, and she moves into a position with a greater international and political focus. She is a central figure in this group, and her intelligence and considerable writing skills lead to even more of an increase in position, salary, and bonuses. She still remains dissatisfied and believes her boss, with no evidence, dislikes her and that she is not appreciated. I remind her that she was convinced her third-grade teacher disliked her when her father became dangerous, and she was terrified of him. She accepts the interpretations with annoyance.

* * *

Her little girl's voice has morphed into the voice of a young but mature woman. She has less ambivalence with her brother and mother. She isolates herself less. She adds healthy foods to her diet, and she starts dating a loving, calm, attractive, intelligent man who wants more than sex.

She feels like she has made a great deal of progress, and decides that psychotherapy takes too much time away from work, and she is feeling ready to stop. We set a termination date, and this phase is emotionally smooth for her. I think to myself that she has internalized our work, our relationship, and the structures of her mind are more suffused with hope, safety, and love. A year later, I am invited to her wedding, where I meet the members of her family, and of course, her biological father is not included.

* * *

*Years pass and I receive a call from Deborah,* who sets up a time to see me. During the first appointment, she tells me that all is fine within her marriage. She tends to be critical in her mind towards her husband, friends, and family members. She knows enough to keep those thoughts and feelings to herself. Her husband is not perfect, but he is loving, a good friend and husband, and she does not want her tendency to be chronically dissatisfied to damage her marriage or other relationships. I think to myself that she has self-awareness and is using this awareness to protect these important relationships.

The problem again is her work. The previous international group she was in, dissolved for political and financial reasons. Her boss was moved to a different position outside of her group. Once again, she was working internationally to help customers use the products. While she recognized the value of this endeavor, she still resented the sales implications of the work. Also, and probably more importantly, she described her new boss as a "bitch." She tells me her boss is demanding, arrogant, not very knowledgeable, and dislikes Deborah. It appears that many colleagues share Deborah's opinion of this woman. An administrative decision is made, and her boss is transferred to another department within the corporation.

With her boss leaving, the leadership of the group is uncertain and other women on this international team are competing for positions. Deborah resents any email that can be construed as diminishing the value of her work. She again starts missing meetings with her departing boss and other meetings. She hides out in her new, beautiful, and expensive home and feels resentful, anxious, angry, and defeated. Her childhood family trauma had organized her child's mind, leading to repetitious behavior: hiding, feeling unwanted, angry, and resentful.

I meet with Deborah and her mother, while her mother is visiting from California. The joint meeting was at the request of both mother and daughter. The sessions are pleasant, and the mother is very loving. Deborah's mother has definite opinions on how frequently her daughter should be meeting with me: three times a week is too much. Her mother also wants to be at the sessions, not to listen and learn, but to convey what the problems are to her daughter and me. Her mother is accurate about a good deal of what she says. I am able to experience how a lack of self-confidence could emerge when "mother knows best" as I listen.

Still, it is vitally important to recognize how this mother came through for her daughter during a childhood crisis. She emotionally and financially supported her daughter, while simultaneously, without her awareness, enhancing Deborah's difficulty with self-confidence and her wish to be protected by a mother-type figure at work. Most of the time these childhood patterns are not too problematic, except when Deborah is dealing with aggressive, competitive, non-empathic women at work. At an unconscious level, the image of these arrogant aggressive women unconsciously becomes connected to the image of her dangerous father and "all-knowing" mother. She goes into avoidant, little girl mode, with the wish to be protected by a loving, powerful maternal figure.

After her mother returns to California, she arrives for her next session and talks about her work with irritation and frustration. "I didn't go to that virtual meeting. All my boss does is complain, and if she mentions me, it is in a condescending manner."

"Dealing with aggressive and condescending people through avoidance is a pattern we have looked at many times."

"Yes, I know. I just can't get up the motivation to go. Why does the company allow such behavior? Everybody knows what she's like. How can they keep her on? I have heard they will be moving her to a different department, but I just will not and cannot go to those meetings."

"Yes, like refusing to go with your father, expecting your mother should protect you."

"I just can't go to those meetings. I don't like the work. The other women say hidden, spiteful things about me. What the Hell! How is this allowed?"

"You still want to believe that if you're very nice and sweet, aggression and competition will not come your way. Remember when we worked on your little girl's voice? It appears that you are not comfortable with the aggression of other women. You are looking for a protective, loving mother. You are not comfortable conveying your personal power, making it clear that you are not available to be punched around."

"I don't want to be nasty or come across as angry, like those other women. Why can't I just continue to be pleasant and nice?"

"Being the good girl will not deter aggression from women who are actively competing with you. It appears you have not found your way of being assertive in a manner that is acceptable to you. Not going to meetings is a form of passive aggression, and I haven't seen that work too well for you or others."

* * *

A large corporate reorganization happens, and a number of her colleagues are laid off, as is she.

At first, she welcomes the layoff, because there is a generous severance package, and she no longer needs to deal with her boss and the competition of other women. After a month or so, she realizes she wants to continue working. The two of us carefully examine what work means to her. She decides she wants to stay in the field of helping others acquire current skills for their benefit. She also faces that she wants to be in an influential position, where she can use her writing skills, her administrative experience, and her enjoyment of working with skilled, cooperative colleagues. She begins an extensive job search and finds another prestigious firm where she is again in a similar role of creating and organizing programs for the benefit of others. She accepts her ambition and acknowledges that she must find ways to embrace her power when being nice and empathic isn't enough. Early in our work, she unconsciously saw no difference between being appropriately assertive and being destructively aggressive. And with her identification with the idealized image of her mother, she thought, always knowing the answer should be sufficient to protect her.

She is excited about this new opportunity and feels prepared to stop therapy. I feel the pleasure of working with her and knowing we have accomplished so much. She feels optimistic about her future and her newly acquired ability to work at understanding herself in a manner similar to our working together. She has internalized the psychodynamic process and has the capacity to use her mind to continue our work together.

# Chapter Seven: DAN

DAN AND HIS WIFE Laura arrive at my office for the first visit. They are professionally dressed, attractive, and respectful. Both are well educated and working in their fields. They have been married for a few years and are in their late twenties. After we introduce ourselves, Dan begins talking.

"I'm here because I'm so anxious, especially at work. I have been anxious all my life, even when I was a very small child. At work, I can barely tolerate the intensity of my anxiety. It's interfering with doing my work. I obsess about small details and am having difficulty finishing anything. I've always struggled with self-doubt and it's getting worse."

"That sounds quite difficult. Do you recognize this as something you felt as a child?"

"Yes, I never dated in high school because I was so unsure of myself. I remember going to a friend's birthday party. I couldn't eat the cake in front of the other kids. It was too embarrassing." He pauses and continues, "I excelled academically and was number two in my class. I was a competitive swimmer and did well. I tried baseball, but my vision was not good enough for that."

I looked into his eyes and saw nothing unusual. He probably recognized what I was doing and told me he was wearing contacts.

I was also observing his wife, who did not seem too involved in the discussion. I asked her what her thoughts were regarding her husband's symptoms.

"I don't understand why he is so anxious and doubts himself. He's a great guy, and very smart. I do have a question. I read that psychiatry is not accepting of religion. We are both Christian. Are you going to require my husband to give up his religion for him to feel better? This is the only reason I am here. I want to make sure that his treatment will not undermine our religion and our faith."

I was surprised. No one had ever asked me this question. I was a bit flummoxed, gained my composure, and answered as best I could. "Psychotherapy is not designed to change a person's religious beliefs. Religion can be core to a person's identity. Core to how they understand themselves and life. A person has a relationship with their religion and their God. This is highly personal. Still, we look at all important relationships, including parents, siblings, spouses, children, work, and religion. The goal is for Dan to understand himself, and this will modify some aspects of his relationships. The primary relationship we will be exploring is your husband's relationship with himself."

"So, you are not anti-religion like Freud?"

"My work is to help an individual understand themselves and their understanding of their world."

Laura appears satisfied that I am not anti-religion. Over the years, I have come to understand how valuable religion can be for religious individuals who are struggling with depression, addictions, and paralyzing self-doubt. The concepts of goodness, a loving God, and the Golden Rule can help render life meaningful when an individual is struggling with emotional distress.

* * *

We meet again, only Dan comes by himself. His wife, Laura, had one concern and was satisfied with my answer and approach.

Dan walks into my office, sits down, and begins talking. “I don’t have adequate words to describe what I am experiencing. I can barely get out of bed. I am so anxious. I worry about the dumbest details. My heart is racing and my palms are sweating as I drive to work. My wife and I plan on starting a family. We both want to have three children. I doubt if I’m capable of dealing with one child. I’m a mess. Will medication help? My family doctor placed me on Ritalin since my mind is so scattered, but it’s not helping. I’ve started doing repetitious things like opening and closing the door, making and remaking the bed. I keep going over the same problem in my mind, over and over again.”

“Yes, I think medication will help. I know your family doctor had your best interest in mind. She was thinking that Ritalin helps calm and organize hyperactive children. I think shifting to other categories of medication is worth trying. You appear to have an anxiety disorder, with obsessive-compulsive patterns. Let’s start with a low dose of a minor benzodiazepine tranquilizer to help calm you. I also want to begin a low dose of a medication called fluvoxamine. It is specifically designed for people with your symptoms. It’s a selective serotonin reuptake inhibitor (SSRI) antidepressant, like Prozac, but with a more specific symptom target. I’ll have you take the medications before bed, and we’ll see how it goes. Are you taking any other medications? Do you have any other medical problems you are aware of?”

“My family doctor says I’m medically fine, except for my psychological symptoms. She referred me to you. Yes, let’s give the medications a try.”

“Okay, I’ll write the prescriptions now. I also recommend meeting four times per week, given the intensity of your symptoms. You have a highly technical career and you want to start a family. You already have a full life, and being psychologically able to stay with your lifelong plans is worth the extra time to deal with your symptoms."

* * *

The following week, we meet and arrange ongoing appointment times for psychoanalysis. I also checked to see how the medication was affecting him. He tells me he is starting to feel calmer, less anxious, and is obsessing less. Over the next few months, I tapered him off the benzodiazepine tranquilizer and increased the fluvoxamine to therapeutic levels. He tolerates the medication without side effects and he will remain on this medication.

During our first few meetings, I could tell that looking at me, face to face, was inhibiting him. He struggles with embarrassment, and I thought he would feel freer to speak to what is on his mind if he were laying on the couch, not looking at me. This does not work for all patients, but it definitely worked for Dan. He was more able to talk freely with me being out of sight. Also, meeting four times per week provided a safe and very available analytic relationship for him to express how terrified he felt. His terror and obsessional symptoms were undermining his lifelong plans for his career and family. He felt paralyzed.

Dan begins to talk more about his life.

"I graduated from college with honors and then went to the California Institute of Technology to get my Ph.D. I couldn't decide on a research topic, so I joined my professor's research team. I wasn't that interested in the subject. I also realized I only needed a Ph.D. if I wanted to teach at a university. I decided I didn't want an academic life. I wanted to be out in the industry. I wanted to build, discover, and advance my field.

"My wife and I met, courted, and fell in love. She actively

pursued me. I doubt I would have had the courage to do the pursuing. She is smart, pretty, and she has the same values as mine. We both want a family. We wanted to get going with our lives, not spend years with me pursuing a Ph.D. I did an extensive job search and received a number of offers. I found the job I have now in Seattle. I knew it would be a great fit for me. My work has been highly technical, involving complicated math and physics. I love the work and goals of this company."

He then tells me in tremendous detail the concepts and the technical aspects of his current project. "Isn't it interesting that I chose a profession where vision is so important when my vision is so poor?"

The session ends and I think about his comments about his vision.

* * *

At our next meeting, I ask him about his vision. "You have mentioned a number of times about your vision being so poor. Please tell me more about this."

"I have severe, very severe myopia. I was born with it. It was not diagnosed until about age three or four. I remember the first time I wore my glasses. I was four. I could see. I wasn't blind, but I hated the glasses. They were coke-bottle glasses. The lenses had to be thick because my myopia was so severe. I hated wearing them. They made me look like a freak. My three older brothers and kids at school would tease me. I felt ugly. I knew no girl would have an interest in me. I joined the swim team because my vision was not that important in the water. I did feel vulnerable when I was walking around the swimming pool without my glasses. I really am blind without wearing my glasses."

"Yes, it is interesting that you would choose work that is so visual."

"The strangest thing is that I'm a visual learner. I excelled in math and the sciences. I think my brain is just wired that way. I feel I can literally see the math, the design, and the physics of my work. I am not an auditory learner. I couldn't do your job. You listen and think. While I look and think. I always wanted to be a pilot, but my mother told me my poor vision would not allow it. I'm sure she was right, but I was devastated."

I now felt I had some understanding of his symptoms. Being nearly blind would have affected his capacity to form a solid visual representation of his mother or anyone in his family. As a small child, he would easily feel lost and would need to follow his siblings. He was actively competitive with his brothers while at the same time very dependent on them, literally following them. He would gloat when he could read sooner than they did or when his grades were better. He compensated with the feelings that he had an inferior body by competing and winning. His feeling of superiority had adaptive aspects. He was able to proceed in life with some self-esteem. This adaptation also leads to considerable emotional and behavioral problems.

* * *

Dan's mother had a severe addiction to sweets. She hid enormous amounts of candy all over the house. His three brothers and sister found and ate the candy, and were overweight, except for Dan. Along with competitive swimming, he had joined the cross-country running team and was very slender. He felt proud of his physique, and he quietly lorded his physicality over his brothers, who were overweight.

He compensated for feeling inferior, as represented to him by his thick glasses, by excelling, especially academically. He believed he was unattractive to girls and never risked dating. He did not trust himself to lead, in any situation, since his vision was so poor. His fear of leading was replicated in the workplace, where his anxiety made making important decisions difficult, and sometimes impossible. His obsessive thinking was probably connected to what he needed to do as a toddler. Without glasses, he needed to memorize where objects were, as any nearly blind child would do.

He often talked about his fear of not being able to see, of becoming lost. “I was driving to a new lab, and I almost had a panic attack. Why would that stir up my fear? There was nothing to it. I got there, calmed down, and the meeting went well. Why?”

“I think your brain was remembering what it was like for you when you were a small child and didn’t have glasses and couldn’t see, especially going somewhere new, on your own.”

“Do you think that could actually be going on? I know I can see well enough to drive. I am correctable to 20/20, so it doesn’t make sense.”

“It isn’t logical, but it is human. There are parts of our brain that remember and record especially stressful or upsetting events. These events are recorded in parts of the brain that are not connected to the conscious parts of our brain. The emotional, out of your awareness, part of your brain is saying ‘danger-danger’. The conscious part of your brain is saying, ‘What the hell is going on’?”

“That is really interesting. Could this be the cause of all my symptoms?”

“If it were only that simple. And, yes, your blindness as an infant and toddler has had an emotional impact on you.”

This dialogue leads to months of exploration and understanding.

“I have always thought of myself as impaired, and not measuring up to other guys. I’m afraid to go to new places on my own. Even when the girls were clearly showing an interest in me, I couldn't believe it. I believed I was ugly with my glasses. I once went to a birthday party, but I was so nervous that I stood in the back of the room. When it was time to celebrate and eat the cake, I was unable to do it. I was too embarrassed and held back. I'm still afraid to try new things because I will look stupid, especially in my own eyes. I panicked over setting up the arrangements for the staff lunch because I felt I didn't know how to do it."

* * *

During the end of the first year of our work together, I scheduled a couple of weeks out of the office for vacation.

Dan describes his dream. "I am driving with my family on a vacation. We are preparing to cross into Canada, and the vehicle I am following vanishes. I panic and wake up with anxiety."

"You know, I will be gone for two weeks. This stimulates some fear in you. In the dream, you are following and panicked when I am out of sight. Didn't you tell me when you left your hometown and went to graduate school, you frequently called your father looking for advice and direction?"

"Yes, I did. I felt I needed his guidance. I felt very alone. My roommate thought it was unusual for me to be calling my father so often for advice. You know, I wanted to be a math professor like my father. I guess I wanted to follow my father."

* * *

We start his second year of psychoanalysis.

He begins a session by saying, "I was playing the guitar last night. I'm pretty good, and I have fantasies of being famous and playing in front of huge crowds who adore me. I know this won't happen, but it's a daydream I frequently have when I'm playing music. That's just like me, isn't it? I do something well and then I want to be the best."

"You are becoming more and more aware of what goes through your mind. I think we both know this is the standard you hold yourself to: 'I'm the best, I win'!"

"It's true. When I was a child, I always wanted to be smarter, stronger, and faster than my brothers. Looking back, this was ridiculous. I was the youngest. There was no way I could be stronger or faster than they were, but that's what I wanted. At work, a colleague was presenting a new digital version of measuring equipment. He did a good job and understood the principles well. I was envious. I wanted the role of being the one who presented our work. I can be such a jerk. Luckily, I understood what I was feeling and kept it to myself."

He stops speaking for a few minutes and continues.

"I am getting bored with all this technical stuff at work. I know it is important, but I end up working alone in the lab, doing nothing but calculations. Where is the glory in that? I've decided to apply to be the new lab director. I have some years of experience and I think I will be a top applicant."

"Moving from technology to an administrative position is quite a rapid change."

"Yes, I know. This is how you advance in the company. There isn't much of an increase in salary, but there is more recognition and more influence. I think my self-confidence is better and I am less worried about making decisions on my own."

"This might be a healthy expression of your wish to be recognized, to join in eating the birthday cake, instead of receding to the back of the room."

"I hope so. I am going to apply for the position. My wish to be the best, to win the competition, is something I need to stay aware of. I'm finishing the classes I'm taking on investing. I've been learning about being an active trader with options. I'm one of the best in the class, but I need to be careful. I must not place our savings at risk. My plan is to only invest ten percent out of one of my retirement accounts. I know I want to be wealthy. I want to be the wealthiest member of my family. My brother is a fiduciary and I want to be richer than him. Yes, I must watch out for this in me."

"Maybe pursuing management in such a technical company might be a healthy solution. Satisfy the wish for recognition and also take reality into consideration."

"Yes, but I know myself. I want to cut corners, and get what I want fast. This is occurring with investing. I have established strict guidelines for myself, but I don't always follow them. I want to believe that my hunches are always correct. Sometimes they are, but not always."

I am impressed with his understanding of himself and how he is analyzing his mind.

At a later meeting, he tells me, "I applied for the job as director and got the job. Now I'm feeling a bit anxious, but I reassure myself with the knowledge that I've been in this lab for a number of years. I am ready."

* * *

During his final year of analysis, his mother dies in her sixties, secondary to complications from obesity. His oldest brother also dies secondary to severe alcoholism. His sadness is appropriate, and he takes all of this in stride.

His children are born and growing, and he is a very involved father. He enjoys being a father and makes a conscious decision to be a fun, kind father, different from his critical, demanding, lecturing father. Life is going well for him and we both agree that stopping his psychoanalysis makes sense. He knows I will need to see him twice a year to manage his medication and to assess how he is doing.

* * *

*Decades have passed,* and he is now in his late fifties. His decision to go into management has worked out well. To his surprise, he enjoys helping colleagues who report to him. He believes that he learned some skills from our work together, and he is now quite adept at working with his colleagues. His children are doing well, are in college, and his marriage remains loving and supportive.

Unfortunately, he is now obese. When I first met him, he probably weighed about 170 pounds. Now he weighs about 270 pounds. He tries to rationalize this by saying everybody in his family is large, except his father. His father was upset by Dan's weight gain and, during a recent visit, tried to lecture him about taking better care of himself.

We meet and talk about his weight gain.

I say, "You have said you are obese, and then you explain it away by saying everybody in your family is like this. Have you developed any medical problems?"

"Yes, but I doubt they are related to my weight gain. I have sleep apnea and use a CPAP machine at night. My family doctor said I have developed diabetes and I'm on medication for my blood sugar. Oh yes, I have hypertension. This is all just a part of aging, isn't it? You're slender like my father and you probably have medical problems, given your age."

"Dan, this is very serious. Your mother and your brother died young, and that is where you are headed. All of your medical conditions are probably caused or made worse by your obesity. If you want to live a long life and enjoy your family and everything you have worked for, we better get back to work. I am deeply concerned. We need to understand what emotional issues are driving this self-destructive behavior. Let's return to using the couch since it does help you to more comfortably explore the deeper aspects of your mind. Given all the gains from our previous work, and especially your capacity for self-awareness, I think twice a week will work fine."

"I know you are correct. I know I have been fooling myself. I'm not sure why I'm doing it."

"You have told me your mother was angry with your father for all his lecturing. You also told me she hid candy throughout the house, and all the kids would find the candy, eat it, and gain weight. You and I have thoroughly analyzed your identification with your father, and how you will act in an arrogant manner like him at times. You have worked very hard to not replicate that pattern. Now we are looking at another pattern you are replicating."

"Are you saying that I am acting like my mother? She didn't give a damn. She did what she wanted! It made my father really angry, but he could do nothing about it. His lecturing had no impact. She ate what she wanted. My brother drank what he wanted. No matter how angry my father got, they did what they wanted. Okay, I will agree to meet twice a week."

* * *

We continue to talk about his weight gain and his pattern of sneaking during the next session.

"So, tell me what you know about your eating patterns."

"I love to sneak in food when my wife is not looking or aware. I'll go to the grocery store and to keep my wife from knowing, I'll pay with cash to buy bakery goods and other sweets. I think it's just as important to me to be able to sneak around to get it, as it is to eat it. I get a real kick out of the sneaking."

"Like a little kid?"

"Yeah, I did that a lot as a child. I'd go into my brothers' bedrooms and sneak out something to annoy them. I was the little one, so they weren't allowed to beat me up. I've always been a bit of a sneak and a tease. I get to work late, all the time. My manager told me it sets a poor example, but I keep doing it. I'll waste time on my iPhone in the morning instead of going to work. I'm not sure I will be able to turn this around."

* * *

A month passes, and he has avoided talking about his weight.

"You haven't mentioned your weight. You talk about your sneaking patterns and how you truly enjoy being a little kid who is a sneak, but nothing about your weight."

"I'm continuing to gain weight. I'm up to over 275 pounds. This is probably hopeless. My blood sugar is up and my blood pressure is climbing. My physician has increased my medications."

"You have a food addiction, primarily with sweets. You haven't mentioned alcohol, is something going on there?"

"I love sweet alcohol drinks. I can drink half a bottle of Kailua and other sweet drinks. I haven't mentioned it because I feel ashamed. I know better, but I don't seem able to stop myself."

"We are going to have to shift our approach to your therapy. This is very serious and you are going to die or have a stroke. You and I must work together. Has it occurred to you that you are expressing your anger towards me as a father substitute?"

"No, I don't think I'm doing that. I just can't stop myself. I don't think this is about you."

"Of course, this is complicated. Your childhood, your mother's patterns, your father's anger, and your brother's alcoholism and early death are all involved. Today, the two people who are truly most involved with you are your wife and me. How do you think I feel when I know you are destroying yourself?"

"My wife is very concerned. She has offered to not buy any sweets for the house. Or because we have young adult kids, she said we could lock the sweets up, and I would be the only one who would not have a key. She says she doesn't want to lose me. She is worried about my health. I guess you probably have similar feelings. You are also worried, and probably angry at me for what I've done."

"Helpless anger is what you want me to feel, just like your mother wanted your father to experience. Your mother wanted revenge and chose something that rendered your father helpless. Your brother was an alcoholic and was angry with your father when he died."

"I don't know about my getting revenge on you as a stand-in for my father. It is worth thinking about, but that understanding will not deter me. Believe me, I know myself."

"I think we need help. There are numerous programs for weight loss. Given that you are a numbers guy, and given that I know there are measurements to deal with this type of addiction, perhaps you could assess the available programs. As long as you share the measurements with me, and you value the program, then I expect this will work."

* * *

He returns the following week and we continue our discussion.

He says, with guarded optimism, "There is a program that tracks your activity level, weight, BMI, diet, and calories. They have an office close to you and I can go there right before my appointments with you. I'm going to give it a try. Is that it or do we do something more?"

"Yes, you and I will observe the patterns you have outlined, namely your sneaking behavior. I don't think we understand those behaviors well enough. Could you still be feeling angry with me as your analyst-father?"

"Okay, I know I'll want to go to Starbucks after this appointment and treat myself. I've been doing this for a long time.

I'm still using cash to sneak sweets so my wife won't know."

"We know you were the little boy in your home. You had a lot of frustration because you couldn't physically compete with your brothers. You also had a great deal of frustration because of your poor vision."

"You think I'm feeling frustrated and feel I am at disadvantage? I think this is more about work. I feel that way at work. I don't feel appreciated. And I don't like my work assignments. I enjoy being a mentor to my younger colleagues, but not all the administrative detail crap I have to read and implement. Lately, I've been feeling that I want to retire. I will have been with the company for thirty years. My pension plan is well funded, and we have enough money to retire. Both of us want to return to Wisconsin. We would be close to our families, and we have already bought a lot on a lake and are working with an architect."

"So, your frustration is with work. You don't like the type of work you are being assigned."

"There are so many things I'm angry and frustrated about. You get these so-called systems administrators who disrupt well-established protocols designed to produce a safer and better product. They come along and tell us that our staffing is too expensive and our procedures take too long and are too expensive. I'm a capitalist. I understand the importance of our stock price, but these people are demolishing the structure of the company, and horrible things have already happened. I'm fed up. I want out."

* * *

Another month passes. He continues to talk about his anger.

"You were right. I have been angry, but not at you. I'm angry with my company. I have been the one feeling the helpless rage. The whole country, especially here in Seattle, is going nuts deconstructing everything. These young people come along. They have learned some so-called new management theory in graduate school. They believe in their social systems theory, and they view disruptions as evidence that their theories are working. The more disruption we experience, the prouder they are. They actually believe this crap. I've had it and I want out." He's quiet. "Oh, by the way, I've lost weight this month. I am not sneaking food. My wife has all the sweets locked up, and I've stopped drinking those sweet drinks. Maybe this has been about me being angry and feeling mistreated by my company."

* * *

Six months later, he has given his notice and announced his retirement from work.

"I gave my notice, and I'm working with my financial advisor to set up a budget for retirement. When I told my team at work, some of them cried. They said they couldn't handle all this without me. I was touched. One woman was so upset she began to sob. I guess I must have been reasonably good at creating trust and respect. I've got to admit, I've learned a lot from you and our work together. It made me a better manager. Oh, I've lost twenty-five pounds."

* * *

We meet the following week, and he tells me about a fainting episode.

"I don't know what is wrong with me, but I fainted while in church. They said I was jerking around. I was out of it. It's probably my anxiety about retiring."

"You are taking medication to lower your blood sugar and blood pressure. All of these medications were started when you were around 270 pounds. You have lost about 30 pounds, and your medications must be watched carefully."

"No, I think it is just anxiety, but I will go to my doctor today and have my labs checked. How could 30 pounds make such a difference? I'll do it, but I think it is a waste of time."

At the next session, Dan reports that indeed his blood sugar was low around 60 mg and, his blood pressure had dropped considerably. He continues with his weight loss program. His weight loss also continued to lower his blood pressure and blood glucose levels. He still does not want to believe his changing lab values and blood pressure are connected to his weight loss. He remains committed to the weight loss program. Within about nine months, he weighed 180 pounds, 10 pounds above his weight, when I first met him in his late twenties. He continues to have fainting spells, once while driving. His physician finally stopped all diabetes and blood pressure medications. His CPAP mask is adjusted to the smaller size of his face. He feels more energetic, and no longer has diabetes or hypertension.

I think it was so difficult for this intelligent, data-driven man to accept the obvious. He had to admit that what he was doing with his addictive eating was destroying his body. What is most important is that he is now healthy, and is no longer in medical danger. His diet is sugar-free and alcohol-free, and he is now walking and doing other exercises daily. He had relinquished his passive-aggressive, masochistic revenge by self-destruction, a pattern he obtained via identification with his mother.

From Dan's perspective, facing and openly feeling his intense anger at the unnecessary chaos created by the administration at work made it possible for him to express and then let go of his anger. He understands his self-destructive eating as an expression of his helpless anger at work and understands that this form of expressing anger is a family pattern, first introduced by his mother. Clearly, he and I would not have been able to accomplish this rather amazing change if he were not involved with the effective weight loss program that included weekly measurements and dietary education. Also, only with a form of psychodynamic therapy that leads to his understanding his out of awareness motivations and resentment would such an excellent result be accomplished. Both forms of treatment, a cognitive-behavioral weight loss program, and psychodynamic psychotherapy were necessary to deal with this life-threatening addiction.

* * *

He has now been retired for about a month and is trying to determine what he will do with himself. He attends church daily and started proselytizing to his children. One daughter, who is more liberal, said she could understand a young woman obtaining medication to stop a pregnancy at the very earliest stage. He went into a rant. He went on and on with anger.

After he finished describing the interaction, I comment, "You can permanently damage your relationship with your daughter and your other adult children by acting in that manner. To go on a moral rant is exactly what your father did with you and other members of your family. Unless you apologize to your daughter, she will feel resentment as you did with your father. This needs to be repaired."

He understands and later tells me, "This morning my daughter called me to try to make things okay between us. She did not say she was wrong. She said that she did not want differences of opinion to come between us because she loves me so much. I apologized to her and said we should have the freedom to have a difference of opinion, even on such a moral issue, like abortion. She did remind me she was only talking about the morning-after pill."

"You no longer have your professional position as an expert. It is not too surprising that you are unconsciously looking for areas of expertise. You want the respect and the careful listening you used to have at work. You've been studying your religion and maybe you've slipped into the role of a moral expert without being aware of it."

"I have been thinking about possibly working part-time, maybe after we move to Wisconsin. Dealing with the architect and general contractor for the house we are building is not as easy as I thought it would be. I'm definitely not an expert in that field, and I do feel unsure of myself. What you're saying makes sense that I still want to be an expert in some area. Maybe being a docent regarding the civil war, or a docent in my field at a science and industry museum might do it. I might return to my field part-time. It's quite a vacuum to fill. Working full time as an international expert to being retired and an expert in nothing is difficult. I never considered that aspect of retirement."

He paused, and with a child-like grin says, "You're retiring in a couple of months. What are you going to do? Are you going to write a book? Will I be in it? Come on, you can tell me." Dan laughs and looks at me

"I am dealing with similar issues. That's probably why I recognized it so quickly in you. It's quite a shift, and it's a journey we will both be taking."

* * *

We continued to meet until I retired. He did not regress or feel resentful. I think he felt ready.

He spent the remainder of our time creating in his mind their new house under construction, reminiscing about our work together, and his thoughts about how to replace the feeling of importance and relevance he had with his work. He did wonder whether the pandemic with virtual communication and in-person masking had an impact on the way he felt about work. Still, he was certain that it was time for him to move on, with work, with therapy, and with Seattle.

# Chapter Eight: DENNIS

DENNIS, A THIRTY-TWO-YEAR-OLD MAN, requested a referral for his emotional distress from the human resources department of his company. He calls my office, sets up an appointment, and we meet for the first time. He is tall, maybe around 6' 6". His height-weight ratio is appropriate, and he looks strong. He has a beard and a full head of red hair. He has never been in psychotherapy and seems at a loss as to what to say.

I ask him, "How might I help you?"

"I don't know. I think I'm unhappy. I don't know what is wrong."

"Tell me about being unhappy."

"I don't know, but I'm alone most of the time. I'm not very good with people. I've always been a nerdy type of guy. I really don't know."

"Maybe if you tell me some details about your life, I'll get an idea of what you are experiencing."

"Okay, I work at—." He abruptly stops, remembering that his company's human resource department had referred him to me.

"Oh, you know where I work. Anyway, I'm a programmer and have been working on this new program function that has been widely successful, making lots of money for the company. I'm already wealthy by my standards. No one in my family has the amount of money I have. I'm careful investing my money since I know the stock market is volatile, and not too predictable. I majored in math and did well enough, but not well enough, to get a Ph.D. Advanced math is way too theoretical for me. I took to programming easily, and I'm quite good at it, and can even be a bit creative." He stops again, looks slightly embarrassed, and shifts around in his chair. "By my family's standards, I am widely successful, but I don't feel that way about myself. I watch a lot of pornography and can see my penis is too small."

"You're a large man, and this can affect the way your penis appears to you. A regular size penis on a large body can appear small."

"I've measured it, and it is only about three inches long. That is small."

"Three inches when erect?"

"I've never measured it when I have an erection."

"It looks like you're a tall, strong man who feels small. Out of your confusion, you measure your not-erect penis and prove to yourself that you are a small man. Do you tend to feel that you don't have what women want?"

"Oh yeah, in all ways. I feel like I don't have what anybody wants, male or female. I need to be careful with my money because I know people want money. To be honest, I'm not sure I trust your interest in me. My insurance pays you and my copay is reasonable. But I suspect that you are in it for the money."

"Maybe you have difficulty believing that more than money motivates me and you."

"Money doesn't do it for me anymore, now that I have quite a bit. Yes, you are correct. I do wonder, all the time, what motivates people? I feel little motivation."

The hour is nearly up and I ask him about meeting again. "We need to stop for today. Will this time work for you next week?"

"Yeah, any day or time works for me. I work alone most of the time and have a fairly flexible schedule."

After the session, I think that he is quite an emotionally constricted person and not comfortable talking about himself. He is not psychologically minded, his self-esteem is poor, and he doesn't have a solid feeling of himself as a man.

* * *

The following week, we meet for the second time.

He looks uncomfortable and says, "What should I talk about?"

"Whatever is on your mind."

"I need more than that. I need some guidance."

"You talk about being lonely. Are you dating anyone?"

"I have a girlfriend, and we meet off and on. It's sexual, but I can't tell if she is very interested in sex or in me. She keeps to herself. We work at the same company, but we're in different departments. She's not very tall. She likes sex, but then she disappears for days. Maybe she leaves town, but she never tells me where she is. It's like she runs hot and cold. She says very little and English is her second language. She grew up in Mumbai, India. We're not that close. I don't know. I don't know if I want the relationship to last. I don't know."

"Dennis, these are the main impressions I have so far about you. You are lonely and feel at a loss of what to do. You don't appear to enjoy your work, and it seems you don't know what to do about that. You struggle with considerable self-doubt."

"Yes, that is all correct. But what do I do about it? I have no idea of what I should do."

"In my experience, somebody with these problems, with a long history of success at school, college, and work, most likely has the ability to benefit from psychoanalysis. This means we will meet four times per week, and if all goes well, you will form a trusting relationship with me and together we will explore your difficulties. The goal is for you to understand yourself and to work on your emotional conflicts."

"Okay, I'll do it, but are you doing this for the money?"

"It's hard for you to believe that I could have a genuine interest in you. I'll call your human resources department to get approval from your insurance company. Your company is very supportive of employees receiving psychotherapy."

He agrees to meet four times per week. Since he feels so lost, I understand that he will require some guidance from me. I can already tell he is looking for a parental figure to guide him. I decided to provide some of this, in the beginning; otherwise, the process might never start.

* * *

He walks into my office and lies down on the couch. I am again impressed by how tall he is.

"This couch is on the small side. My feet are over the end. Well, that's okay. What should I talk about, and please don't ask me what is on my mind?"

"In order for us to understand you, we need to explore your present-day relationships, your experience of yourself when you are alone, and your childhood. Your relationships with your parents, siblings, and so forth."

To my surprise, he starts talking openly about his childhood, and we spend the next few months exploring his early life.

"I love my mother. She is smart, was the main breadwinner, and worked as a teacher and as an auditor. She loves me, I know that, but she says very little. She's a bit of a loner.

"Both of my parents are deeply religious, and my father insisted I attend a religious high school. The school was okay, but it was not where I wanted to go. I wanted to go to public school, but my father won, and I did what I was told. I was really angry with him most of the time. My mother was the smart one. My father worked as a non-skilled laborer, mostly as a janitor for the public school system. He would yell and scream at me and at other people. We recently went to dinner, just the three of us, and of course I paid. At the end of dinner, he made a few religious comments to the waitress. He made her and me uncomfortable. I keenly dislike him.

"He'd drink at least a bottle of wine every night and, after dinner, he would give me stupid instructions about what I should do with myself. He tried to give me instructions on how to have sex with a girl. He told me I should play around and have lots of sex. I hated his lectures. But if I objected, he would yell and scream and have a temper tantrum. It was easier to sit there and appear to be listening to this dumb, drunk man who was supposed to act like a father."

I interpret, "Your difficult relationship with your father might have contributed to your confusion about how to feel about yourself, especially as a man. Even though you are tall and strong, you feel small and weak."

"I saw a picture of myself with my girlfriend and her friends. I couldn't believe how large I was. You are right. The way I feel about myself and my body does not match my reality."

* * *

The next week, he begins to explore his relationship with his mother.

Again, he is uncomfortable and asks, "What should I talk about?"

"Your description of your father and how you feel about him is rather clear in my mind. Your mother, and your relationship with her, is not as clear to me."

"My mother is rather quiet. I'm pretty sure that she is angry with my father, but she would never say that. Why would she marry a man so much less intelligent than her? Why does she stay with him? Maybe it's their religion. I know I tried to be the son who would please her. I know she enjoys my intelligence and my academic and financial success. I never act angry like my father. I never drink excessively. I don't needlessly argue with people. I am not like my father. I'm glad about that."

"Frequently the son, especially an only child like you, will move closer to his father to figure out how to be a man, and how to psychologically separate from his mother. Given your father's actions and drunkenness, you would not or could not listen to him. I think you turned towards your mother for guidance on how to be a man, and in general, what type of person to be. This had to have been massively confusing for you."

"How could I view my father as an example of how to be? My mother didn't respect him. I didn't respect him."

"And now, you don't respect yourself or trust your own self-direction."

"Oh, I see. My only choice was to be a mama's boy," he says with sarcasm. "Except my mother was never clear about what she wanted, even for herself. Hmm. You're saying this is where my confusion about myself started. I never thought of that, even though it is obvious once you say it." He becomes quiet and pensive.

"I was with my girlfriend and wanted to initiate sex. I couldn't tell what she wanted, and I was not about to force myself on her, the way my father suggested. He said that women do not know what they want sexually, so you just need to proceed. It doesn't look like that worked so well with my mother. She is fat. And I get the impression she does not want to be touched. When I hug her, it's never a full hug, more like a polite hug. I know she loves me. I can tell. I paid for their kitchen to be remodeled. It was expensive. She sent me the bill with a note thanking me and saying she loves me. Damn her. There it is. I have to spend money to get clear verbal assurance that I am loved."

For the remainder of the year, we focus on his hatred of his drunken, religious, fanatic father, who he refuses to be like. He also is quite sure that his mother only tolerates his father and does not love him. We also explore how he is always trying to get a read on what his mother wants of him. Given that she is a rather hidden person, he is, out of his awareness, continuously scanning her for approval. He is beginning to understand that this is his pattern with women.

* * *

We begin his second year of analysis.

"I don't like my work anymore. I've made my money and I don't like the isolation. Since I was one of the main inventors of this program, I have nothing more to prove. I don't need the money. Why am I staying at work?"

"As we both now understand, following your own lead, as to who you are and what you want, has been problematic for you most of your life."

"I have this problem in relationships with women. I don't know what I want, so I follow their lead. My girlfriend doesn't act like a girlfriend. She disappears for a week, and then never tells me where she's been. I'm sick of putting up with that, but if I bring it up, she talks about leaving. I don't know what to do."

"It's clear to you that you keenly dislike her pattern of disappearing. Do you tend to think this is how she feels about you? Or is this just the way she is, and she would be this way with anyone she is involved with?"

"Oh, I'm definitely taking it personally. What you're saying never occurred to me. That she could just be this way, and it has little to do with me. That's a good point. Why couldn't my father have had that type of understanding and wisdom?"

* * *

Dennis stops seeing his girlfriend. He starts using some dating sites and joins a few dating groups. Much to his surprise, he enjoys himself and feels that most of the people he meets like him. He had a few sexual encounters but does not form an emotionally close relationship. He appears to be doing what he wants, which is dating and having fun.

He discusses at great length how he feels about his work. He changes his position at work and becomes even more isolated. He decides he wants to leave the company and pursue something else. He feels a little guilt and shame at no longer working, but not too much. For over a decade, he worked ten- or twelve-hour shifts until the program he helped create was completed. It was wildly successful. He became wealthy, and he wants out.

Within the paternal transference, he is not looking for my approval. In the maternal transference, he concludes that his grueling work and wealth have given him the right to do as he wishes. I view all of this as progress. He understands himself better. He is better able to emotionally connect with himself, and he is feeling, for the first time in his life, independent. He is an independent person who now knows what he wants. My role is that of an analytic developmental parental object that understands, is emotionally present, and neither approves nor disapproves. This analytic process results in enhanced self-cohesion and capacity for self-reflection.

* * *

As we begin his third year of analysis, he has blossomed. He leaves his company and buys an expensive house. He is actively involved in remodeling the house and plans to buy a second home in the mountains. He is dating, investing, and not looking for my approval. I am aware that my role is to be present and aware of what he is feeling and the meaning to him of his actions and decisions: an emotional mirror. He no longer talks about having a small penis, and he recognizes that some women will want to be with him and others will not. I give no advice or opinions. I understand that his finding his psychological independence is new and wonderful for him; I must not interfere.

He meets a professional woman in a nearby city. They fall in love, and he decides to move in with her. I talk with them both on the telephone. She is in therapy and will continue with her therapist. If problems arise in their relationship, she wants to consult with her therapist. Dennis and I have one more in-person session. He is grateful for how I helped him. He is ready to stop.

This is not how I conceptualize a psychoanalytic ending, but who am I to question such a change? He is delighted. They plan on having a family, and he wants to be actively involved in raising the children. I know he is moving through separation, individuation, with parental object removal as an emotional adolescent with me. It's sort of like, "Well, I'm moving out, going to live in a different city. I've found the love of my life and we are going to have a family. Oh, and you, dad, keep your mouth shut." Like Dennis, I am also delighted with his growth and maturing self-understanding.

# Chapter Nine: MARK

THE HUMAN MIND is the most complicated entity in our world. We have complex brain and mind functions that will probably be explored, studied, and modified until the end of our time. Whether to proceed with psychodynamic psychotherapy is a very complicated and vital decision. When both the patient and the psychotherapist agree to proceed with the psychodynamic process, another important and complicated decision remains: whether to convert or not to psychoanalysis.

I chose the case of Mark to provide more clinical details regarding the therapeutic process of psychodynamic psychotherapy and the question of conversion to psychoanalysis. My hope is to provide a more in-depth understanding of the process of psychodynamic psychotherapy and psychoanalysis. Two human minds, working together, trying to understand the emotional suffering of another, is a fascinating, massively complex, emotionally engaging venture. Providing more detail with this psychodynamic process may help in understanding how an individual can benefit, and why being a psychodynamic psychotherapist or psychoanalyst is a lifetime journey of learning.

* * *

Mark walks into my office, introduces himself, and floods the session with details about how he was referred to me, his current and previous employment, and his past therapy experiences.

"Dr. Furedy, I'm Mark and was referred to you by Dr. Smith. I wanted to see him because he knows my New York City psychoanalyst, but his schedule was full. You know, I just moved here after I was fired from my hospital position in New York. I joined a group of anesthesiologists and I got my assignment at Good Samaritan Hospital almost immediately. I'm glad I found you, but I'm concerned this might not work. I don't know you.

"The first psychiatrist I saw in medical school told me I would only find peace if I accepted Jesus into my heart. I fired him. A few years later, I tried working with a psychoanalyst. He was quite active, gave some very good advice, and told me my life would not get better if I insisted on being so arrogant." He briefly paused and continued, "I was benefiting from working with him, but unfortunately, he developed horrible headaches, ended up with glioblastoma, and died. I was devastated, felt lost and depressed. I started seeing another psychoanalyst, who was very quiet, took copious notes, said little, and I gained little, if any, benefit. I was seeing him when I was fired from my job. He was of no help."

"So, I'm the fourth psychiatrist you have seen. And only one was helpful, and he died. It takes courage to risk it again."

"I'm so miserable. I don't feel I have much of a choice."

"Tell me about the misery."

"My life is shit. I came to the West Coast with my wife and son and daughter. After a few months, my wife returned to New York, filed for divorce, and accused me of desertion. I'm enraged. What a bitch! I love my children, and I try to talk with them by phone, but that doesn't satisfy me. I do have two weeklong summer visitations with them. I miss them. I'm lonely. I have no friends. And I hate my boss, who is a woman."

"Things have not gone well for you. What are you doing to cope?"

"I drink a bottle of wine every night. Alcohol numbs the pain in some ways. This isn't like me. I have to take a tranquilizer every night to sleep. I'm definitely depressed. I'm angry, anxious, constantly agitated, and I isolate myself. I find no pleasure in my work as an anesthesiologist. I have no friends, no girlfriend. I have nothing. I frequently think about suicide. I'm a mess."

"You are in emotional trouble. Given the crisis you are experiencing, and your familiarity with psychoanalysis, I'd recommend we return to analysis. Would you be able to meet four times a week?"

"NO," he says with considerable anger and insistence. "I am not going to repeat what I had with my last analyst. I will sit up. We will meet face-to-face, and you will be active and tell me what to do like my first analyst who actually helped me. I need help. I need advice. For God's sake, man, don't you understand this?"

I think to myself, establishing trust and a working alliance will not be easy. I feel a bit intimidated by his take-charge demeanor, and have the impulse to refer him to another psychiatrist-psychoanalyst. I know he is going to be difficult. I also know he is in a crisis, potentially suicidal, and I have a moral and medical responsibility to him. In addition, I know that all of his frustration with his last analyst is being transferred onto me, along with his trust and hope for help from his first analyst. I remind myself to be a bit more active than I usually am, since he definitely needs to feel me, and hear me.

I say, "Mark, using your judgment and prior experience, how frequently do you believe we should meet?" I am aware that I am starting the process of building an alliance, where we work and decide together.

"Twice a week should be sufficient, and you will need to be flexible with your schedule since medical emergencies do occur."

"Let's look at our schedules and arrange the times. I understand that you do not want me to be quiet and passive. I appreciate your concerns. I need to inform you that I conceptualize our work as our working together to understand you and your experiences."

"Okay, I'll see you next Tuesday, and don't you dare go silent on me."

* * *

Mark returns to my office for his second session.

"My boss, Dr. Ray, is a woman. Did I tell you that? She has all these crazy ideas on how we should run the unit. She insists that my concerns about the lack of adequate assessment and evaluation of patients before I start to anesthetize them are not relevant. Can you imagine that? We are physicians and we should be making these decisions. Who in the hell does she think she is? I told her off. I confronted her and my colleagues were all quiet. They're wimps. No wonder I didn't discuss this issue with them. They're all stupid wimps."

"You feel a lack of support from your colleagues who you believe cannot understand. Do you think it is possible that the intensity of your rage and feeling abandoned became worse when your wife and children left you and returned to New York?"

"Yes, I've always had trouble tolerating ignorance and passivity. And you're right. I am angrier since I lost my family. How could she do that to me? Then she accuses me of abandoning them in New York when she was the one who refused to live out here. What a bitch! I've never had a comfortable, loving relationship with any woman. I'm not very good with women."

I am cautiously trying to establish a trusting alliance by empathically mirroring his angry despair, and at a minimal level, introducing the concept of displacement of feelings from one person or situation to another.

* * *

Mark returns for his third session. "You think I am getting rid of my anger at my wife by directing it toward Dr. Ray?" he asks.

This was encouraging. He clearly understood the meaning of my comments and has been thinking about this. I don't answer his question directly. Instead, I say, "I notice that you feel you can't trust your colleagues and that you need to address these crucial issues on your own."

"Hell, I've felt that way my entire life. I have two older brothers and an older sister, and they were never any help. They teased me, and all I could do was kick them. When I was in graduate school, I did well, received my Ph.D. in chemistry within four years, and joined the faculty. The department chair would not listen to my ideas. He was not receptive to new, more advanced ideas or innovative programs, and the faculty did not support me. I became so angry. Finally, I became so frustrated that I decided to go to medical school and specialize in anesthesiology. I figured that if I were a physician with a Ph.D. in chemistry, people would listen to me. I would have the authority, the knowledge, and would be taken seriously and admired.

"You must tell me what I should do with Dr. Ray. This should never be allowed. Patients are sent to me without basic lab work or a thorough physical exam. I can't anesthetize them without basic lab work and a physical exam."

Again, I direct his thinking towards his colleagues. "You know this issue is of vital importance and I notice you do not seek out your colleagues as a potential source of support as reasonable thinkers. It's like you must do this on your own, similar to the way you described your experiences with your older brothers and sister."

"What do my siblings have to do with my situation at the hospital?"

"For reasons that are unclear to me, I think we may be looking at a pattern that developed during your childhood when you concluded that others were of no help."

"My siblings didn't give a shit about me. Look, I was diagnosed with childhood rickets when I was three or four. It was severe. The doctor diagnosed a vitamin D deficiency; probably because of the unhealthy food my mother fed me. So, they put me in leg braces. They would place me on the sun porch of our house to get maximum sun. I wore braces until I was fourteen years old.

"I felt loved and cared for when my parents took me to see my doctor. He was wonderful, a man ahead of his time. Under his care, I had a full recovery, but I was in braces until I was fourteen. When I was not in my braces, I was confined to my bed, since my legs and hips could not support my body. My mother was a chronically unhappy, angry, unloving woman who took me to the bathroom when I needed to pee or defecate. She was the only one who took care of me. I think she resented my illness, requiring her to attend to me more than her other children.

"I couldn't go outside to run with the other children. When the doctor said I no longer needed the braces, I was so glad. I also missed the feeling of security I had with them. I could use them as a weapon to kick my brothers. Again, what does this have to do with my problems with Dr. Ray?"

I interpret, "You know, the careless assessment of patients before being anesthetized is a serious problem. You came to understand that your rickets was a serious problem and, if not treated properly, would cripple you. You concluded that your siblings did not care about you and, therefore were of no use. Only by the guidance of your family physician, and the care of your parents, were you able to become able-bodied. The helplessness and frustration you felt then, and your conclusion that your siblings were of no help and were useless, has some similarity to how you are feeling now: alone, no physician in charge to protect you, and no trust or help from your siblings/colleagues."

"I'll think about that. It is almost too much to digest. None of my other therapists ever mentioned my rickets and braces. This hospital problem is serious. No hospital should allow ER physicians to admit patients to surgery without a complete evaluation. No hospital should operate in this manner. You keep suggesting I should talk with the other anesthesiologists. Hmm."

"Your experience with your family physician had a profound impact on you. He's the type of physician you want to be: a man before his time, respected, who can relieve suffering. Some of your medical ideals for yourself are connected to your profound experience with him."

"I never thought of that. It makes sense. I can feel how accurate that is. I did think that my superior knowledge of chemistry would give me a leg up in the competition with other anesthesiologists. I want respect and admiration."

I decide not to further explore his other references to his childhood, since there will be plenty of opportunities later. I have already given him an enormous amount to think about. I don't want to overload him. I am also concerned he might be experiencing me as dismissing or explaining away his genuine present-day concerns by referring everything back to his childhood.

* * *

The following week we meet, and Mark describes his interaction with his colleagues.

"I met with the other anesthesiologists and, to my surprise, they agreed and we met with Dr. Ray. I could tell she was annoyed, but she agreed to discuss this issue with the ER staff. I took the lead with the other physicians, and tried not to be too arrogant like my first analyst told me."

He spends the remaining time in the session venting about the ignorance of the hospital administration. Toward the end of the session, he says, "God, I wish I had a girlfriend. I may be forty-nine, but I'm really horny."

I thought he might be beginning to trust me. My understanding of his concerns regarding the hospital problems and referencing his older siblings, perhaps, is reminding him of positive feelings toward his first analyst. He spends the remainder of the week describing how devastated he was to lose his children, but not his wife. He never loved her, nor did he respect her very much. He felt his importance to her was the money he brought home.

* * *

After the weekend separation, we resume our work.

"I was thinking. I've never been in love. I think of sex as a biological need, and that women should understand and stop making such a big deal about it. It's nothing more than just body parts that need discharge."

"You have never been in love? What about high school or college crushes?"

"No, never. I was always about achieving good grades and winning any competition I entered. The person I loved the most was my father. When I was young, I worshiped him. I could ride on his strong shoulders, and he was proud of me, especially my intelligence. He was an impressive man, educated, intelligent, and successful. He had three businesses and made a lot of money. He was also deeply religious. When speaking, he sounded like a preacher and I loved listening to him. With hindsight, he was very dogmatic and suffered fools poorly. He was in charge at home, and my mother's job was to do whatever he demanded. When I was twelve, they divorced. My father moved to another city in the same state. He made no attempt to maintain a relationship with me or any of his children. It was like he had just moved on and forgotten about us. We were no longer of any importance to him.

"My mother was an angry person, even before the divorce. When I had my leg braces, she did take care of me, but I could tell she was angry. She was angry all the time, and so I concluded she was angry with me. When I left home for college, I was glad to get away from her, and from my brothers and sister.

"My father, even though he lived in a nearby town, never came around or showed any interest in us. Months before he died, I took him out of the nursing home in a wheelchair and rolled him to a remote location. We were alone. He couldn't speak. He had Alzheimer's. I spent a couple of hours screaming at him for what he had done. How he had abandoned us, his self-righteousness, preaching, and everything else I could think of that I was angry and disappointed about. I felt better and took him back to the nursing home. I did not attend his funeral."

I respond, "Maybe somewhere in your mind, you decided loving was too risky. You could be abandoned. Your wife leaving you and taking your children might have touched on the pain of being abandoned by your father, and confirmed loving is dangerous and people are not to be trusted."

"Yes, that makes sense."

* * *

Even though Mark is able to integrate my interpretations, having benefited some from his previous psychoanalysis, he routinely misses about one session every two weeks. When I inquire about this pattern, he says that his previous analysts understood that he is a physician working in a hospital, and medical emergencies take precedence over his treatment. He believes his previous psychoanalysts understood, accepted, and never questioned his absences. Having treated other hospital-based physicians, who practically always made their appointments, I suspected there was more to this, and maybe his previous psychoanalysts had indulged him instead of exploring and interpreting. I also wonder if this might be me being competitive.

After seven months of psychotherapy, he returns to my original recommendation for four times per week psychoanalysis, given he can see he is feeling better, and making some progress. Also, this is likely evidence that I have passed his evaluation of me, that I would not be passive like his second analyst.

He says, "Why not take full advantage of psychoanalysis? You still need to accept that there will be times when I will be required to attend to a patient in immediate need."

We establish appointment times that should not interfere with his work. The very next week, he cancels two appointments. I am annoyed and realize this pattern should be analyzed.

When he returns, I say, "You canceled two appointments last week. What happened?"

"You know how hospitals are. Things come up."

"So, what came up?"

"At the request of another anesthesiologist, the scheduler decided to change my shift. Why are you asking me about this? This is just a hospital reality."

"Missing about one-third of your appointments will interfere with what we can accomplish. Why would the scheduler place you on that shift?"

"Why wouldn't she? She has no idea of my appointment times. I don't want to get on her bad side."

"So, you are telling me that you have never revealed your current or past therapy appointment times?"

"The scheduler is a woman and I am not comfortable telling her my schedule for analysis. You know how women are? She'd probably tell everybody in the unit and embarrass me. They will all think I'm a weenie. When she asks me to do something, I say yes without thinking. I do this with all women. Eventually, my resentment becomes so great I explode with anger at the woman I am obeying."

"This is a pattern you have in your relationship with women you need. You are afraid to tell her your schedule because you expect some form of angry psychological attack. With your mother, you needed her to know when you needed to defecate or pee, but I doubt you would tell her. You waited for her to figure it out, and I think you may be doing this with most of your relationships with women."

"You know, this might make some sense. I would get furious with my wife when she did not appreciate how hungry I was, especially when dinner was late. I've never told any woman, with words, what I want sexually. The scheduler should know by now how much emotional trouble I am having. Why should I have to tell her? She should know. I do not want to tell her I'm in psychoanalysis four times per week. I'll try to talk to her, but it will be difficult for me. I don't want her to think of me as an emotional cripple."

"I think you believed, because of your braces, that your siblings and kids at school would see you as weak, as a cripple. You might think of psychoanalysis as helping to brace you up."

"Yeah, you're right. I felt ashamed of my weakness as a child and I feel ashamed now. When I was out of the braces and could run, I was proud. I think my father understood that. My legs became very strong. Did I tell you I'm thinking of buying a mountain bike and riding it to work and our sessions?"

He decides to buy a mountain bike and comes to his sessions in cycling shorts, which revealed his strong muscular legs. I did comment on his pride in his body, especially the healthy strength of his legs and hips.

He keeps most of his appointments after talking with the surgical scheduler. He comments that my body build reminds him of his older brother. A memory comes forward of his older brother holding a sword over him when he is awakened from sleep. He is not sure if this is a memory or a dream, but he can easily see he was afraid of a physical attack from this brother. When he was a teenager, they had a few physical fights.

I comment, "These memories coming forward today probably indicate that you have some fear of being on the couch and my being behind you."

"Yes, it is a bit creepy with me being in a vulnerable position and not being able to see you. In high school, I was wrestling a guy in a match. He pinned me and won the match. I was infuriated and my anger and adrenaline strengthened me and I threw him off of me, put him in an armlock, and then broke his arm. I got into a lot of trouble because of that. So yeah, I'd prefer to be able to see you. This is dumb. I know that you are not going to attack me, but all of this comes to mind."

I think that even though Mark is frightened, he is already free-associating and self-analyzing. These are strong indicators that analysis is the treatment of choice for him. Also, he is able, sometimes, to distinguish the reality of me from his transference of me as a dangerous older brother.

* * *

The analytic sessions are filled with details of his external problems, leading to his suffering and justifiable rage. When I interpret that his inner world is organizing his experience of his external world, he feels criticized, surprised, and disappointed. He wants advice from me on how to improve his life for the better.

I interpret, "You want me to be the brilliant father who carries you on his shoulders, and can give you lectures about right and wrong."

He responds with confusion and protests, "I didn't come here to explore my relationship with you. I came here for advice."

* * *

After about six months of psychoanalysis, he is calmer, seems to feel safer with me, no longer uses a tranquilizer, and drinks wine only in moderate amounts. His panic and temper outbursts have decreased in frequency. This is consistent with establishing a positive early parental transference, creating a feeling of being held with a background of safety. It can also be understood as establishing a mirror transference that is stabilizing his narcissistic equilibrium.

By a mirror transference I mean that my capacity to see him as he is, to understand what he is feeling, and putting this into words, and correctly understanding his emotional conflicts, I can provide for him an emotional mirror, a relationship where he can see himself, as I explain what I see and understand. This leads to a self-representation that is different from before. He experiences himself within the relationship with me, and this modifies his self-representation. This analytic process also alters his experience of me. I cease being the competitive older brother holding a sword over his head. I become someone he can trust, which generalizes to his emotional view of others. Some people can be trusted. He does not have to always go it alone to be safe.

He is quite intellectual and views me as unusually perceptive. At times my interpretations are too wordy and intellectual. I think this is my unconscious response to actualizing the idealized early-father transference. When he pressures me for advice, I sometimes unconsciously comply. During the sessions, I usually think I'm "in the moment." It is not until after the sessions that I realize I was giving advice.

He has a strong wish for a strong, wise early father, and out of my awareness, at those moments, I feel and become and act like the wise early father he lost. I am lost in the moment, and the nonverbal intuitive aspects of my mind are influencing my thinking and reactions. He senses me and I sense him. This is an intersubjective process. My subjectivity, most of which is nonverbal and emotional, interacts with a similar process in him. We both respond to this nonverbal, intuitive process with words, actions, emotions, and co-created understanding.

* * *

With time, he moves on to an awareness that he acts like his father, who abandoned him when he was twelve, and he struggles against his identification.

"All of what comes out of me is bad: my humor, actions, thoughts, and feelings. I am unacceptable. I'm just like my father. My mother said he was crazy. He could not maintain his business or his family. I'm going to fail just like him. My father would proselytize all the time. Unfortunately, I'm doing the same about proper medical practices. When I catch myself acting like him, I feel ashamed and humiliated. When I fly into a rage, as he did, I feel humiliated and disgusted with myself."

I quietly interpret, "Maybe you identify and act like your father to feel as if he is still with you to avoid the pain of his abandoning you."

"You know, I act like I'm suffering because my wife left me. That's not accurate. I wanted the marriage to end. This is another example of me acting like my father. He was always claiming to be suffering at the hands of others."

* * *

His regression to an early childhood transference, organized around his braces, total dependency, and painful enemas emerged during the middle of the second year of his analysis. He is very concerned about losing control of himself and others. He is afraid of being overwhelmed and unable to control his feelings and bodily sensations. He voices his concern that I will invade his mind and take control.

"You know, I'm somewhat paranoid. My first analyst would tell me I'm forever showing my asshole to the world, putting my worst foot forward."

"Maybe you are experiencing a fear and a wish that I take control of you and your body like you experienced with your parents as a small child unable to care for yourself."

His immediate associations are to memories of his parent's preoccupations with enemas. "If I didn't feel well, my mother gave me an enema, which frequently hurt. I also remember early times with my mother, that were warm and comfortable. I remember feeling her breasts against me as warm and comforting. I am a weenie. I'll do almost anything to please a woman. No matter how silly their wishes, I comply."

I suggest, "Perhaps being in bondage is a way of feeling close to a woman and me as your analyst-mother."

"I always feel in harness. Bondage is a way of life for me. I can't tell the medical director my schedule. And I can't tell you what my schedule is with the surgical suite. I am in bondage with her and with you."

* * *

As a holiday separation approaches, his defenses against his experience with separation result in his arranging for a two-week vacation before the scheduled holiday separation. I tell him he is leaving me before I leave him, trying to exercise control, and deny my importance to him, since being left is so distressing to him.

After the three-week separation, Mark returns and is frantic. He is unable to lie on the couch. He insists that I change the treatment format and claims he needs advice on how to live his life. I tell him I think he is angry with me for leaving him with overwhelming feelings. He experiences the three-week separation as abandonment.

When he arrives for the next session, he is able to lie on the couch. During the separation, he carried the image of me as angry with him for not paying his entire bill and missing appointments.

He angrily says, "You weren't available, and I went into oblivion."

I understand his anger as separation terror from a parental transference object. He attached his feelings onto an image of me, as angry and rejecting, so in his mind, I had abandoned him. I was nowhere to be found.

He continues, "I felt you were angry with me and I felt rejected, so you weren't emotionally available to me and I felt panicky."

"You couldn't have the feeling I was with you since you believed I was angry with you."

Mark talks about feeling abandoned most of his life, believing nobody really cared about him, feeling truly alone and panicky. He tells me, "It's like falling into a dark abyss, no one to reach out to and no one to hold you."

* * *

Mark continues exploring his experience of being "in braces." For the remainder of the analysis, he uses this metaphor of "in braces" to understand his emotional world. He tries to understand his feeling of something good relating to the braces.

He says, "Braces resulted in my mother, my father, and my doctor showing an interest in me, spending extra time and money on me. Braces were providing me with support. It was painful, and it hurt to walk, but I could also use my braces as a weapon to kick my brothers."

I reconstructed that during the early years of his childhood, he didn't experience himself as healthy and able to separate from his parents and have confidence he could be on his own, and confidence that his mother and father were still loving and available.

He has a dream where he is at the barbershop, receiving a haircut. "New hair. Maybe my mind is growing new hair. Maybe you are trying to help me have different responses. I'm either overly aggressive, trying to control people, or I'm dependent, passive, and in service. You speak to my being "in braces," feeling restricted early in life. It's like I'm in bed, completely dependent, having to be seductive, or racing around aggressively trying to be in total control."

He believes his mother's neglect created the vitamin D deficiency, which resulted in his diagnosis of rickets. "Even then, I blamed her for my rickets. This may have something to do with the helpless rage I feel towards women. When I was in bed, I was one hundred percent dependent on my mother. It was her fault."

I say, "You believe you need to be braced up and supported by people you don't trust, at times with me, and as a child with your mother. To feel braced up, in pain, and helplessly angry are familiar feelings and at times you just go there."

* * *

The second year of his analysis involves continuing to work through his transference with the analyst as an early maternal object. At times, during separations, my failure to exactly understand what he is experiencing disrupts his narcissistic equilibrium. He unconsciously wishes I were a part of him, a self-object, that can know and understand exactly what he is experiencing. At these times, he is painfully confronted with the reality that I am a separate person, not a part of him and under his control. This anger eventually is followed by shame and humiliation, and panic secondary to knowing we are separate. To avoid the pain of separation, he will unconsciously go to his identification with his images of his omnipotent early father. But acting in such a grandiose manner now leads to shame, which motivates him to access his capacity for self-analysis.

This needed repetitious working through results in the maturing of existing intrapsychic structures and also the emergence of a marked change in his affect. He is seldom depressed, has more energy, enjoys and takes pride in his work, and starts dating. At times, he actually seems happy and hopeful. He begins to understand that his life does not have to be a series of experiences where he feels tied to people he does not trust, does not like, but whom he must obey. Maybe he will be able to feel free to run, play, and enjoy himself. He has a dream where he is riding his mountain bike through a new city, exploring and enjoying the new terrain. Both he and I understand this dream is stimulated by his new feelings of freedom with pleasure and excitement.

While analyzing another dream, where he is receiving another haircut, but this time a modern haircut, he quickly understands this as an indirect reference to his analysis. He says, "Analysis has loosened up my superego and I am more able to play and enjoy myself. It might sound to me like you want to control me with your words, but now I understand that this is a collaboration. It's like we're doing research together."

Mark's statement demonstrates his ability to better differentiate the analyst from the parental images he has always carried in his mind. Parental objects that entrap him while wearing braces enter his body with painful enemas, and on whom he is totally dependent. This is a vivid example of how the development of early childhood transference and then analyzing the transference can lead to impressive psychological changes. His mind drifts to a drunkard, Dennis Day, in a recent movie.

He says, "My dreams are so vivid now, like images in an art gallery. I'm so glad I gave up alcohol. I don't need it anymore."

* * *

Near the beginning of his third year of analysis, there is more of a movement away from his anal-sadistic and masochistic (painful controlling or painfully being controlled) infantile wishes and fears, to more phallic wishes to compete and feel like a strong man. When he feels anxious about his conflicting feelings of competition and affection towards his colleagues, he will return to the anal position as a defense against his fears and discomfort with working together, as a team built with respect and affection. He wonders, "Where is the control and strength in this?" He feels the impulse to regress to outrage and the wish to control.

"Where is my protection from attack if I relinquish my rage? When I was wrestling in school, my rage gave me the strength to defeat my opponent. I broke his arm and got into a lot of trouble. If I give up my rage, I'll be like the monks in Tibet or the Anasazi (Ancestral Puebloans) who were defeated by the more aggressive tribes. You are kind and patient, and I know I am still afraid of you. Remember, you remind me of my oldest brother, who held a sword over my head."

He reads Robert Bly's *Iron John: A Book About Men*, and

comments, "The key to the wild man is under the mother's pillow. My father was a wild man. He was a religious fanatic, always on a mission, always preaching. My mother liked me when I served her, fixed food for her, and massaged her feet. She didn't like it when I acted like a typical boy. If the key to masculinity is under the mother's pillow…? Well, my mother wasn't very caring. She resented me. I want a woman who will satisfy me and take care of me. I guess I'm looking for the mother I never had. When a woman frustrates me, it taps into my rage. I don't trust women."

Mark has a dream, and for him, it is depressing. He is on a train fighting with a younger man and he pummels him with his fists. He is teaching this younger man a lesson and is trying to explain this to the man's mother.

I say, "Maybe your dream is a continuing reference to the book *Iron John,* saying you will find your masculinity under your mother's pillow."

"Yeah, the wild man." He falls asleep.

I feel frustrated and believe he is passively waiting on the bed to be fed and toileted, tormenting and teasing me. I am the maternal analyst in his dream. At this moment, he is refusing to find his masculine self by looking under my pillow or identifying with his analyst whom he experiences as kind and patient. Unconsciously, he is being passive-aggressive with the unconscious wish to provoke me. I do feel annoyed. He has, before, spent most of some sessions, saying nothing, especially after successful analytic work involving navigating his daily life. If he relinquishes his arrogance, aggressiveness, how will he be able to protect himself?

* * *

Over the next few months, he analyzes his arrogance and aggressive competition.

"I have always had a sense of knowing what is better, particularly in science. When I try to implement changes, it gets me into a lot of trouble."

"Maybe these missions help you to feel more like your father, more masculine, a way to leave your mother."

"I'm never content. I try to use my medical and scientific knowledge to convince people of the clear need for change. I keep doing it, and others have fits. My new girlfriend doesn't respect my medical training. She values her thinking above mine. I have no authority over the surgical staff. If I don't take charge, I feel weak, like I'm sucking hind teat. At least my father gave me one valuable mission. He wanted to see me educated. You say I'm still in bed, passively sleeping and waiting, but I feel like I have no tools to deal with everyday problems. I want to smash and take control or give up. Even my girlfriend will not follow my instructions." He falls into silence and maybe sleeps.

I interpret, "When you are silent for a considerable time, I think you want to be the passive recipient of my knowledge. You seem reluctant to use your own knowledge of yourself to understand yourself."

"None of this means a hell of a lot to me. What use is this self-understanding?"

He is being resistant and attempting to provoke me to act like his father and, at times, himself.

"I bought a new car and openly negotiated the price with the salesman. Usually, I just accept what they say the price is. I gave a presentation about needed changes at the hospital. I was calm, polite, and political, and my proposal was accepted."

He clearly feels proud of himself. He then calmly negotiates an appropriate time change regarding our sessions.

"I'm concerned about the impact of the analysis on me. I feel like I've lost my mission. I feel sort of lost."

"It's not easy to give up your idea of a mission or a crusade. Regular accomplishments don't feel like this to you. You want to continue your father's crusade with your science and medical knowledge. It's like you can either feel great about yourself or feel like you are nothing."

"This leaves me flat. I get no public recognition. I received more recognition in graduate school for my research. Like the characters in Star Wars, I am looking for extraordinary strength and abilities. Without a mission, I feel weak."

I think and eventually interpret, "You alternate between wanting me to be a caring mother, who is demanding control and servitude from you or representing a powerful male opponent that wishes to defeat you, like with your older brother, and at times with your father. When you embrace the reality that we are actually working together, it pleases and calms you, but also stirs up a feeling of loss." He associates it with another political issue at the hospital that he navigated with finesse.

* * *

Mark develops a capacity for understanding the frustrating administrative problems of his boss, Dr. Ray, and is more able to work with her. He begins to have detailed memories of his early father. The reality was that his father was not continuously supportive. At times, his father was easily angered, critical, and used corporal punishment. He is able to connect these memories of feeling criticized and disappointing a father figure like his analyst and the professors in graduate school.

He begins to accept his lifelong concern of being unfairly blamed as a projection of his own thinking. He criticizes himself in ways that remind him of his father when his father was angry. "Freud would be pleased with this understanding," he says.

He must be reading about psychoanalysis to accurately cite

Freud on Freud's concept that the son can separate and differentiate himself from the mother by identification with his father. According to Freud, this identification will then reside in the son's superego.

As the fourth year of his analysis ends, his material is consistent with the beginning of termination, the ending phase of his analysis.

He has a dream that his analyst is deliberately withholding words of wisdom during a face-to-face interaction. He feels hurt. He says, "I can't figure things out by myself. I feel you understand me better than I understand myself. My progress is slow. I get only one or two ideas from you weekly. I want an IV push. It's frustrating. You share your understanding in metered ways. My analysis has had a profound impact on me. It's somehow built into my unconscious. It enables me to avoid a lot of trouble."

I comment on his awareness of his enhanced abilities resulting from his analytic work and how he is beginning to feel the fear and the wish to separate from me.

"God, I was able to work through the administrative problems at the hospital. I guess the analysis is working. I don't trust myself to turn over the care of myself to me."

* * *

His oldest brother visits and he recognizes traits of his father in both of them. "We are both rigid, critical, and obsessed with right and wrong. A gentle, kind woman can't survive with either of us. My brother is going through a divorce."

I think his capacity for whole object relatedness (the capacity to see the flaws in a love object and still maintain affection and respect) is evolving and present. Aspects of his personality are becoming ego-alien to him. He says, "If I act like a raging bull, like my father, I feel more masculine. I'm becoming bland. I feel impotent. I'm pissed."

I interpret, "You equate analytic movement away from being a raging bull, as you remember your father. At times, you feel analysis is a form of castration as if a man cannot be strong without raging."

* * *

He is now more able to enjoy a loving and spontaneous sexual intimacy with his girlfriend. He catches himself responding to her at times as if she were like his mother. He is pleased with this new understanding. He now understands that she enjoys his masculine capacities, and his ability to be appropriately assertive. She does not try to control him, nor does he try to control her. He believes a strong love is developing between them, a love where who is in control is not so important.

His ego capacity for self-soothing and self-regulation without the use of alcohol or tranquilizers is impressive. There are minor regressions during separations. His most recent material is more about wishes and conflicts regarding being an independent, emotionally strong, competent male, and disconnecting this from archaic grandiosity and omnipotence.

He is better able to gain satisfaction with ordinary daily accomplishments. There is enough critical superego modification so he can have less guilt, be more independent, sexual, assertive, and successful. His intrapsychic structures are less organized by a high titer of anal aggression. This makes it possible for more sublimation, as evidenced by his new hobbies and sports. There is more depth to his autonomous ego functions, allowing for more conflict-free doing, seeing, and understanding.

I actively listen to and accept his awareness of his improvement. He sets a termination date.

"My girlfriend is having some difficulty adjusting to my new independence. I'm proud of my ability to interpret my last dream and use it to talk to her about what was bothering me. That 'aha' feeling you get with understanding a dream. Such a clear picture."

I think that this demonstrates his interest and capacity for self-analysis.

He continues, "Instead of complaining, I come up with solutions. I face and analyze problems."

I tell him, "I agree with your assessment of your progress and the termination date of four months out makes sense."

He wonders how analysis works and says, "I no longer play the role of being handicapped."

I unexpectedly cancel an appointment and he is concerned something is wrong and hopes my health is good. He experiences me more as a real person and less as a transference object. He shows concern about his older brother, who is going through a divorce.

* * *

He has a dream about the ER doctors being jailors and controlling him. The dream switches to an image of farmers harvesting a bountiful crop. He talks about feeling imprisoned by his time-consuming analysis. He says, "All of my life, the only way to leave was to escape."

I interpret, "You're struggling with your wish to harvest your fertile analytic crop mixed in with a wish to stay forever. You deal with your mixed feelings in a way familiar to both you and me. Namely, feeling imprisoned, tied down, with the wish to escape."

He has another dream about a man who has hair like his analyst, who loans him a jackknife. He touches the blade and is cut. The fruit to be cut is bulbous at the end. His thoughts are that he is afraid he cannot handle the knife on his own. Will he be able to handle his self-analysis without hurting himself? The fruit has a phallic look to it and he thinks about wanting sex and his girlfriend being receptive. He wonders if he can handle the analytic knife on his own.

New memories of his mother, appropriately worrying about him when his father was pushing him to work long hours to the point of exhaustion, begin to surface. He realizes she definitely showed her love for him and he did so want her love. I interpret, "You experienced my last few interpretations as showing genuine concern for you, and this surprisingly stimulated memories of similar experiences with your mother."

I think to myself again that he is developing the capacity for whole object relationships in his inner world and present-day relationships. His mother is now flawed and also loving.

In keeping with his enjoyment of whole object relatedness, he wants to know some details about my life. Throughout the analysis, out of his awareness, he only wanted and needed an empathic, correctly mirroring analytic function, not an actual person with flaws. He expressed an interest in knowing my history. Why did I become an analyst? I did not feel in any way pried into or invaded; it all felt appropriate and warm.

He felt pleasure and an interest in his self-analysis and was looking less often to me for understanding. We looked at his pattern of pushing himself to the point of extreme fatigue as an expression of his wish to please me as his analyst-father and to avoid any possible criticism of his analytic accomplishments. He speaks to the impossibility of leaving comfortably. He cannot emotionally conceive of it.

He has a wish-fulfilling dream. In this dream, there is a reunion with his brothers, sister, and the rest of his family. He is sharing the beauty of life with them. He then remembers a second dream where he is being criticized for poor sterile technique and ends up feeling bad about what he is doing.

He speaks to wanting to check in with me now and then, aware of feeling anxious and insecure. "I function better and have calmed down. I feel better, but I'm afraid to jump off the diving board." I speak to how his recent material about entrapment in his analysis is a familiar defense against his wish to stay and avoid his fear of swimming on his own.

"I no longer charge at windmills. To function independently is a fundamental change."

"You are now relying on your not-so-sterile technique." He laughs.

* * *

During the last session, Mark spoke of his greed and that he was not pure. Accepting this helps him feel free to be masculine and know what he wants. Maybe he is freed up from his lifelong concern with guilt and evil. He examines his wish and fantasy that his analyst cannot let him go and realizes that his friendships will not be a substitute for his analysis. This last session is sad for both of us as we say goodbye.

# Chapter Ten: LOOKING BACK

I HAVE PRESENTED eight examples of psychodynamic psychotherapy, sometimes combined with psychoanalysis. These individuals only represent a tiny sample of the people I have attempted to help. Their stories are different, but they all have one thing in common. They were hobbled by the intensity of their painful emotions.

## FIRST STAGE (OPENING PHASE)

Over the years, I have had calls from people who have said they want an appointment because their spouse insists, or they have a court order for treatment, or their human resources department referred them as a requirement from their employer. Under these conditions, the necessary trust and motivation may not be there. Oh, they might set up an appointment, come a few times, and then disappear. Sometimes these individuals might find a self-help group or another therapist who is their choice. What I have learned is that it must be the decision of the patient to pursue treatment.

Unless they find self-motivation, the work will not proceed.

If the individual is openly suicidal or a danger to others and refuses appropriate treatment, involuntary treatment may be required. When I was in my psychiatry residency in Wisconsin, I rotated through Mendota State Hospital. I was asked to see an involuntarily committed patient named Gerald, who was yelling and screaming, and clearly psychotic. When not psychotic and in the hospital, he had a profession and worked full time. When I met him, his speech was too fast, his thinking was too rapid and scrambled, and he was highly emotional. I had read about using a new medication called lithium carbonate to treat bipolar illness, back then referred to as manic-depressive illness. I had no experience with this medication and neither did my supervisor. I talked this over with Gerald and he was willing to give it a try, as was my supervisor. The medication worked, we achieved a therapeutic level, and Gerald was more stable, with a mind no longer racing or consumed with psychotic thoughts.

We discharged him, and I followed him as an outpatient. He greatly appreciated my commitment to him. He returned to work, and he wanted to meet with me weekly to talk about how he was feeling. I was not trained as a psychodynamic psychotherapist, but I did listen and I gave little advice. His wife also joined us during some of his sessions. His bipolar illness had resulted in massive interpersonal problems in their marriage, and they needed help. I obtained supervision; Gerald and his wife worked in couples therapy, calmed down, and were able to achieve some insight. The treatment ended as I was finishing my psychiatry residency.

During the last week of my residency, I saw Gerald sitting in the lobby waiting to see me without an appointment. He was there to say goodbye and wish me luck with my career. A fondness had developed between us, and he was grateful for my commitment, the correct diagnosis, a new and useful medication, and the individual and couples therapy. Life was now better, and he no longer needed to spend half of his life at Mendota State Hospital.

Why does Gerald come to mind? He was psychotic and involuntarily hospitalized, but he invited me in. There are times, under the worst possible conditions, the individual will invite you in. We were lucky that the medication lithium carbonate had just been discovered, and it worked well for him. Even under the worst circumstances, a little magic can happen. Gerald invited me in and we were a good fit. And I knew enough about general psychotherapy and medication to help him. I suspect if we met today, we would still be fond of each other and would get a good chuckle over the time when he was psychotic in the hospital and stuck his naked ass in my face. What a profession!

With hindsight, I was using some of what I learned early in my professional journey from my experiences with the autistic boy Billy and the teenager grieving his mother's death, and from the knowledge of Carl Whitaker and other mentors. I had learned to listen with kindness, not assume I knew what the answer would be, try to establish an emotional connection, and be genuine.

Trust and working alliances are usually achieved as the individual starts to tell you about their worries, their pain, and their ideas about themselves. It is so important to restrain ourselves from jumping in with astute interpretations. Wait, listen, and then, when you believe the individual might be able to understand what you are thinking and seeing, speak. Don't rush. Make the interpretation and listen carefully to their response. Remember, you might be missing the main point. Keep your interpretations connected to present-day conflicts, something like, "When your manager suggested that you should improve in that area, you felt hurt, like she was seeing you as defective, and you wanted to hide." Later on, during the mid-phase of treatment, you can connect the experience to their childhood feelings and conclusions about themselves and their parents.

When I told Dan that sneaking food was revenge on me, like his mother did with his father, he in essence said, "No, not this time!" He did not feel my interpretation was correct. He went on to talk about his deep resentment towards the ridiculous and frustrating changes occurring at work. He resented the foolish decisions that were disrupting decades of his work to make a safe and reliable product. He spoke to me of the self-impressed systems administrators who were disrupting his life and the lives of his employees. They routinely said, "This process takes too long. You don't need so many professionals trained at such an expensive level. Hurry through the process so we can get this to market." He spoke about how their changes could and did, lead to dangerous results. He said, "My reaction to them is more like my reaction to my father. I'm angry, resentful, and feel helpless. Those administrators are acting like self-righteous bastards like my father. It's not about you. It's about the stupidity of the men I report to."

I had made the transference interpretation, which seemed quite obvious to me. I was correct that he was feeling helpless anger and seeking revenge, but I was wrong that it was about the way he felt towards me in the transference. He was able to correct and complete my interpretation. Together, we were working to understand.

Psychodynamic psychotherapy is very much about working together with the patient. It is not about receiving interpretations from the analytic guru.

The way to establish the working alliance, an alliance that will be kept until the end of treatment, is by doing your best to understand what the individual is feeling, especially their emotional pain, the feelings towards family members and others who are emotionally close, and thoughts and feelings about self. If the psychotherapeutic process is internalized, the individual will be able, some of the time, to provide this function for themself. This is called internalizing the therapeutic process. Identifying with the analyst probably will occur, but again out of the individual's awareness. Having the capacity to understand yourself, your common conflicts, especially your patterns for dealing with painful emotions, can become permanent and invaluable.

## SECOND STAGE (MIDDLE PHASE)

Usually, emotional conflicts are unconscious. In this phase of therapy, where the therapist is interpreting to the patient out of awareness emotional phenomena, there is a subtle but important shift in the work. When Mary returned for psychotherapy, there was a shift from emotional mirroring to interpreting unconscious conflicted emotions and behaviors.

I said to Mary, "You are in your late seventies. Your abilities are not the same and this is the main reason you retired. You don't have the same energy you once had. With your volunteer work, you are trying to work at the same pace as you did when you were working full time. Let's explore why this is so important to you. It's important to recognize you are exhausting yourself and you are using anger to discharge all these feelings onto those close to you."

This interpretation is long, but not that complicated. It is rather obvious, but Mary didn't know this. She was surprised. She thought that other people deserved her anger because they were not meeting appropriate standards.

This is an example of needing to interpret a prominent conflict repeatedly. Mary is unable to accept the realistic limitation of herself, secondary to aging. This is such a common problem. You see it in the media. Eighty is the new sixty! Or, sixty is the new forty! Not true.

Mary's frustration with herself is projected onto those around her. When her anger is discharged, she feels calmer for a while, and then it all starts again. This is the type of intervention I can make only after I have been invited in and I am trusted not to criticize. I am not telling her to knock off her ranting. Wrapped into this material and the process, I interpret and she comes to accept that she is acting like her childhood critical mother with whom she has identified with since childhood.

Remember Dennis, who was 6' 6"? I said to him, "You feel like an undesirable man. You isolate yourself and are feeling lonely and resentful. Even though you are big, you feel small, like you're a small man. You avoid the very thing you want most, a loving sexual relationship with a woman." This type of interpretation is only allowed and useful to an individual after the patient and therapist co-create trust, a working alliance, and an emotional connection. Only then were we able to look at how he's turning away, not wanting to be anything like his father, which contributed to his confusion and uncertainty regarding his masculinity.

And with Ted, I said, "You are feeling so anxious and unsure of yourself. You are acting like you learned everything from your previous psychiatrist. I have trouble understanding you because you are performing and are not connected to what you feel or to what you are thinking. This long-standing pattern of performing, trying to impress others, has led to you having little sense of your true self." Nobody would tolerate a stranger, or anyone not trusted or invited in, to say anything close to this.

An analytical space is created through careful, empathic listening that opens up room for exploring together the painful conflicts of the patient. Without careful first phase work, these interpretations would fall on deaf ears and be rendered meaningless. We were able to move into understanding that Ted's father's alcoholic impairment and his mother's anger towards his father led him to always try to be his mother's good boy. He had never individuated from his mother. Instead, he tried to perform to please her and others, and never developed a cohesive sense of himself. This early mid-phase work, empathic mirroring combined with interpreting central emotional conflicts, started the process of the emergence of himself, a man he could respect and take pride and pleasure in being.

It is imperative that the psychodynamic therapist, first and foremost, starts with the patient's current struggles and conflicts. Referring to memories of traumas, childhood conflicts, and transference interpretations will usually come later. Except when it doesn't. Some people will start their work with a childhood trauma/event. Something like, "I have this dream. It's repetitious, and I wake up with a fright. It's something about my older brother and me. It's very upsetting." The therapist at this point is in no position to understand the dream and the childhood events connected to it, but you must start where the individual starts. You wonder, with the patient, what the nightmare might mean. Memories may just emerge. Sometimes, that is just how the mind works and the co-created process emerges

Establishing trust and a working alliance by listening makes it possible, and safe, for emotional material, deeply repressed, to emerge and be analyzed. The safe analytic space, along with the trusting attachment, facilitates the emergence of repressed feelings and memories. Whether they are repressed, denied, or dissociated, childhood or adult trauma will carry intense emotions. These emotions might lead to temporary, therapeutic, psychological regression, which can be quite confusing and frightening for the patient.

Both with Shelly and Deborah, all of this happened. Shelly, who had massive drug abuse problems, was able to recover traumatic memories after she had spent a successful year in psychoanalytic psychotherapy and then psychoanalysis. When she remembered her father allowing his drug dealer to use her sexually as a child, she was devastated, disorganized, and not able to work for a few days. But so much fell into place. She began to be able to put together why she did this and that, and why she chose unreliable men.

When Deborah remembered and accepted the importance of her father's attempt to kill her mother, and his stalking her after school, her fearfulness and childlike presentation became understandable. Recovering these childhood traumas is not the end. It is part of a process of needing catharsis of repressed traumas, and an understanding of the elaborate mechanisms used to adapt to the trauma. These adaptations can be static and lifelong if there is no conscious understanding.

Not all individuals who are dealing with emotional suffering have experienced dramatic childhood traumas at the hands of a parent. The imagination of a child has few limits. Children are capable of creating tremendous emotional conflicts despite having loving and understanding parents. The child might be frustrated and might project these feelings onto a parent and believe that parent is frustrated with them. Or a child might have a physically painful condition, and the parent is unaware or unable to relieve the pain. The child might conclude that the parent is indifferent to their suffering. Being in chronic pain will frequently stimulate aggression and suffuse the mind with anger, which will often be directed towards the parents or the self. This can alter the relationships and or the representation of the parents or the self in the child's mind. If the child is psychotic, he might believe his parents are frightening, dangerous, and not to be trusted.

In another example, the child may have an overwhelming experience outside the home, like a near-death experience with his bike and a car. The child may be overwhelmed, and unable to put into words what happened. The child may start acting up as a way to discharge his intense feelings or as a non-verbal attempt to communicate his experience and emotional state to his parents, who are likely to not understand and become annoyed with his misbehavior.

The child might have been going somewhere that was off-limits, according to the parents. The child is too afraid to tell his parents and also feels guilty because he broke the rules and almost died. The terrifying event, combined with the child's inability to speak, resulting in the child acting up and the parents becoming annoyed, could all be repressed and forgotten. The event is still recorded in parts of the child's brain that do not produce conscious memory but do produce non-verbal procedural memory. As the child matures into adulthood, he, and others, may not be able to understand his confusing actions and feelings.

Creating a safe analytic space, as I have described, provides the potential for remembering, catharsis, and understanding. By recovering these powerful emotional memories, they become conscious and available to the rational mind.

The patient and therapist can now work with the recovered material, leading to possible intrapsychic changes in the mind of the patient. Self-representation, how the patient sees himself, might change. Feelings about family members might change. Career decisions might be affected and feelings about oneself might change. In my experience, most of the individuals I have worked with have had events that overwhelmed them as children. After recovering the memories, working through the intense emotions, understanding the emotional and behavioral patterns that resulted in the response to the trauma, they can make substantial changes.

Both the therapist and the patient can gain access to areas of the mind that are connected to different types of memories. Some neuroscientists will refer to procedural memories, things you do without being aware you are doing them. Others will talk about implicit memories, memories that are not attached to words or consciousness. Freud referred to these memories as unconscious memories.

There is active research in the areas of procedural and implicit memories. Multiple areas of the brain are being explored, and as the research proceeds, a depth of understanding is accruing. This research may become an integral part of the evolution of additional treatments for emotional suffering, especially in childhood and adult trauma.

From a clinical perspective, it may be useful to think of the brain as having two memory systems, conscious and not conscious. The conscious memories also involve multiple structures of the brain, including the prefrontal cortex, with the capacity for abstract, critical, and creative thinking. It is complicated, much more complicated than this brief explanation. What is most important to understand is that there are brain anatomic reasons why humans can be so unaware of so much of what they remember or what they do.

Do you remember when and where you obtained your accent? Are you aware you have an accent? Yes, this is a ridiculous question, but try speaking with a Scottish or an Australian accent. Intellectually you get it, but when you open your mouth to speak, you are not in control of or aware of your accent. This is a small example of how much of what we do, feel, say, and act is out of our awareness. An accent could be referred to as procedural memory, completely out of your awareness, unless you are motivated to change your accent, and engage in a process that facilitates an ongoing conscious awareness of your accent.

Our reality is that so much of what we do and feel is not under our control. That is where the deepening of the psychodynamic process comes into play. The process leads to our becoming aware of ways we respond, think, feel, behave, and talk in areas that need to be addressed because they are creating trouble for us or causing emotional suffering. That's why you recover the unconscious. It is imperative that you go back into childhood or previous adult traumas, to see what happened, how to understand how you adapted, and to understand that you may still be thinking, feeling, understanding, responding, and behaving similarly as when these overwhelming events occurred.

This is not just about recovering from the horrible things that are done to children. Sometimes, that is exactly what happens. Other times, it is decisions or adaptations that a child or adult makes, again, out of their awareness. The eight stories I have shared demonstrate, during the mid-phase of treatment, how psychodynamic recovery and healthy modifications of emotional and behavioral patterns are possible.

Mark started therapy, believing that his responses, thinking, emotions, and actions were all logical and appropriate to his colleagues at the hospital. He had no idea that he was displacing his anger toward his ex-wife onto his female boss. He did not understand that having rickets and being in braces led to feeling helpless, feeling he would always be a cripple, and then proving to himself and others that he was not a cripple, but superior. He cycled for miles in his bike shorts to reassure himself how strong he was, and to reveal to others, and me, the healthy musculature of his legs and body.

Mark did not understand that after his father abandoned his family, he kept his father around by acting like and identifying with his father. He did not know that he was doing medical proselytizing, just like his father did with religion. He did not know that he acted like a know-it-all, using his Ph.D. and M.D. to prove to himself that he did know it all. He understood none of this, but as we uncovered and explored how he was now replicating his father's behavior, he was able to accept and start modifying his actions.

Mark also did not understand the way he responded to women was similar to the way he experienced his mother. Since he was in present-day psychological braces, women should know what he needed without him needing to say anything. He could not trust any woman's deep love for him, as he misinterpreted his mother's anger. Instead, he would revert to being very passive and expect to be taken care of without ever needing to say a word. The unconscious painful memories of being "in braces" were operating as procedural memory, directing his feelings and actions towards women, with poor results. As he understood and remembered all of his "in braces" experiences and how he was replicating this now, he began to alter his way of relating to women, eventually resulting in a loving and enjoyable relationship with his girlfriend.

Ted had no idea that he had developed a false self. His work with me deepened after his job, marriage, and child-care legal realities were dealt with, and as his trust strengthened in me. He came to understand and accept how his father's drunken incompetence and his mother's rage led him to feel it was unsafe to become his own masculine person. He adapted by disconnecting from his sad, frightening feelings by performing. It was not about enjoying academics; it was all about acting as if he enjoyed learning to receive applause, good grades, and his mother and aunt's approval. He was not aware of liking or enjoying his sport, but wanted his coach and mother to watch and praise him without criticism. With no competent father to identify with, or help him psychologically individuate from his mother, he became an actor, without knowing that was what he was doing.

Our mid-phase work was about him attempting to generate opinions or approval from me as a parental figure. Left on his own, he went into performance mode, which did not work well. Instead, it led to feeling intense anxiety and a lack of awareness of his thinking and feelings. The more I correctly mirrored his emotions and thinking, the more he could see, hear, and feel himself. This did build an experience of self. He discovered so many aspects of himself: his type of movies, music, intellectual interests, work, and the appearance and personality of women he found appealing.

When he began dating, Ted was performing, assessing how well he had done and was not tuned in to how he felt about the woman. This also changed with insight, when he recognized that he was not sure he ever wanted to form a lasting monogamous relationship with any woman, because all his previous relationships with women had been about his acting to please and doing or not doing what he was told. Again, none of this was conscious until we dove deep into his childhood experiences and analyzed how these patterns were in place during his marriage and now with dating. It was difficult for him to reveal that he wanted to have fun and play. In his maternal transference to me, he expected I would want and believe he should do what I had done and get married. This is an example of how transference emerges and can be interpreted and accepted by the patient. After the analytic process has deepened, the patient has the opportunity to understand how he is responding to the analyst in patterns similar to central childhood figures.

## ENDINGS

People end their work and therapeutic relationship in different ways. As with all other phases of psychodynamic psychotherapy, the ending of therapy has a different complexity of meaning for each individual.

When Dennis found a woman he respected, wanted to marry,

and have a family, he assumed our work was over. He had accomplished what he desired. Saying thanks and goodbye to me was a release, freedom for him. I represented, in his transference to me, his religious, unhappy, controlling parents. He just left and moved to a different city. He wanted separation. He wanted the excitement of being in love, and the adventure without his religious parents looking over his shoulder.

With Dan, he kept a connection with me throughout the years, partly because of medication management, and also because he did not want to leave his father-analyst. As I was retiring, he was retiring. He actively used our capacity to work together to understand how he used food as an expression of anger. He rendered me, in the paternal transference, helpless by damaging his body, as his mother had done with his father. His addictive eating was much more complicated than that, and we needed an external weight management program to provide monitoring. The sneaking of food was a lifelong compulsive behavior, and we needed external help to resolve it. Left to his own devices, he was not able to control himself; it was a compulsion.

Each week, he reported the results of his measurements, and there was no hiding from that. Of course, if the trust and genuine relationship had not been in place, he could have undermined any program. Dan wanted to remain the youngest, nearly blind, special member, of his family. Sneaking, annoying, making members of his family of origin so frustrated and helpless was just too enticing. Our work led to him finally accepting that he was seriously damaging his body, and placing his wife in an impossible position, which was not acceptable to him. He needed the relationship with me to understand what he was doing, and to accept his need to relinquish this pleasurable defiance.

Dan and I were both looking at retirement. He longed again to be the smartest one in the family and started using religion, like his father, to become the superior one. This too, dissolved upon analysis. Demeaning his daughter about a moral issue is not being religious; it is about the wish to be superior. This also changed with the analysis.

Dan kept working on himself up to the end of his psychotherapy. He most likely was consciously thinking that it was now or never: "If I want to deal with my compulsive eating and sneaking, I better do it now while my therapist is still available." One can see his self-awareness and his ability to constructively face the reality of the ending work. He was aware of the impact on him of our ending and used it to finish his work.

The wish to be brilliant had created problems in the past for Dan. We explored the idea of his finding enjoyment in pursuing areas of his interest, not to prove himself superior, but for the enjoyment of the work, and the pleasure of being with colleagues. He was quite sure he could find part-time work in his field, especially with such high demand. We were both disappointed that we had to end our work virtually, but the pandemic was more powerful than either his or my grandiosity.

Mary was angry about my retirement. She did not understand that her demands were unrealistic. She demanded to see me in person, and I reminded her of the masking and other COVID-19 requirements in a physician's office. She argued that she met with friends and family, and did not need to wear a mask or take other precautions.

Later that week, she went to her family physician's office for a routine visit and also volunteered at a local hospital. At the next session, she apologized and said she knew better. She acknowledged there were Washington State and CDC requirements for any physician's office. She went on to say this was just like her, as we had discussed all year. She does not like frustrating reality and will become angry and criticize others for not doing the correct thing. She now accepts that she has identified with her angry, critical, arrogant mother and is using this response when she is scared or frustrated. We continued working in therapy up until my final retirement date.

Ken and his wife, Jennifer, took the ending in their stride. They had each other and could work together to continue the psychodynamic process. About a year before I retired, Ken had hired a business coach that he thought would help him with his feelings, thinking, and approach to real estate development. I looked at the coach's website, and he described himself as more like a therapist, but he had no training. Ken had paid a considerable amount of money in advance to retain the coach's services. Ken tended to be impatient and impulsive. We discussed Ken's decision during a session. He recognized that he was feeling at a loss with my upcoming retirement and thought this could be a replacement. His wife and I, along with the business coach, after he obtained some of the details, all questioned Ken's decision. Ken was able to understand that he never had an available parent, especially an analyst-father like me, and must have wanted a replacement. He understood and canceled the contract with the business coach. It was sad for all three of us to end our work together.

Ted's response to my retirement announcement was emotional dissociation, as if it were not happening until he set a date to stop. He regressed, became childlike, and took a week off work, because he correctly assessed he should not be working, given the complexity and importance of his position. He understood that my retirement was a reliving of his parents' divorce when he lost his father. He understood that the feelings were so intense that he disconnected himself. He stayed with a younger female cousin for a few days for emotional support. Staying with her was an advancement, in that he always portrayed himself as the emotionally strong one that she came to for support. He relinquished that role and analyzed his intense feelings about our ending work.

After his weeklong therapeutic regression, he returned to work and made arrangements to see one of my female colleagues. He understood he needed to work on his considerable distrust of women. The regression was so intense because of the dissociative mechanisms he had used throughout his life.

Both Ted and I marveled at how much he had changed, from being the passive, anxious, hidden boy-like man, to being a leader at his company, managing his finances, dating, knowing who he is, and feeling pride and having knowledge and access to his emotional world.

Shelly's psychoanalysis occurred years before my retirement. At that time, she was working in her field, dating a man she loved and was ready to finish her psychoanalysis. She understood the impact her father's orchestration of her childhood rape and betrayal had had on her. She realized she was using drugs to not feel, not remember, and not re-experience the danger and terror of the traumas. We ended our work together fondly. I attended her wedding, and years later, she brought her child to my office and requested her baby blanket back. She understood that asking me to keep her blanket safe in my office was a way to feel part of her was still with me. Now she was ready to take that part of her back as we said goodbye.

Deborah was ready to stop treatment and prepared for my retirement. We worked through so many issues. The one remaining issue had been her fear and hiding when dealing with competitive women who were plentiful in her field. In time, she obtained another job more consistent with her professional goals. She understood her passive hiding pattern of dealing with aggression had not worked for her, and she was focused on not repeating that pattern with her new employer. She felt ready, and I experienced her as ready. Her marriage was comforting, loving, and stable. The goodbye was sad. Some months later, she sent me a book featuring short poems based on the author's childhood memories. I understood the book as a goodbye gift and also a nod to accepting that her childhood experiences with her father were of immense importance in understanding her symptoms.

Mark finished his work with me years before my retirement. He felt ready to stop. He dropped by my office once to say hello. He also sent me a delicious apple pie sharing his hobby of baking with me. He was no longer in conflict with colleagues at work. His romantic relationship with his girlfriend became permanent. He made summer arrangements to be with his three children. We had a calm, rewarding, and fond ending.

* * *

As I look back over the many years of working with individuals, I am reminded how privileged I have been to be invited into the inner world of so many because of my profession. Being invited in is an essential aspect of psychodynamic psychotherapy. Being invited in does not always happen. For an individual to be talking openly, trying not to censure their thinking or what they are saying is quite a leap of faith. Even though formal meetings end, the work does not. Each individual will consciously, and unconsciously, remember the understanding, will re-experience our working together, and will explore their inner world with curiosity and less guilt and shame.

# RESOURCES

## TREATMENT

Psychodynamic psychotherapy is not the treatment of choice for all diagnostic categories. Also, the process has little appeal for some individuals. One size never fits all. Since you have just read this book, you now have some understanding of psychodynamic psychotherapy. Does it appeal to you? Can you comprehend how this approach might work for you? If so, it could be life-altering.

How do you find the right therapist? Not all mental health professionals are therapists. And not all therapists are trained as psychodynamic psychotherapists. Do your research.

The American Psychoanalytic Association's website (www.apsa.org) can assist you in locating trained psychodynamic psychotherapists and psychoanalysts throughout the country. The psychoanalytic institute in your city or nearby is another excellent resource. Their websites can help you find a well-trained psychodynamic psychotherapist. Today, many clinicians have their practice-related websites and will often describe the concepts they use while working with individuals.

Once you have decided to start psychotherapy, make an

appointment. The demand is very high secondary, to the virus and the continuous growth of the virtual world. This growth has increased the number of people who are vulnerable to feeling isolated, lonely, and disconnected. Do not get discouraged if you are unable to make an appointment immediately. If the therapist you call is unable to see you because of scheduling issues, ask if they can recommend another therapist who might have open times in their schedule. It may take time, but you will find someone with the skills you need.

Once you set up an appointment, trust your intuitive sense of the fit between you and the therapist. The work is a partnership: two people working together to understand the mind of the one who is suffering.

## TRAINING AND CONTINUING EDUCATION

Psychodynamic psychotherapy training is available for individuals beginning their professional careers and to seasoned clinicians wishing to expand their knowledge. Your local psychoanalytic institute and the American Psychoanalytic Association (www.apsa.org) websites can assist you in finding training programs at psychoanalytic institutes in your city or nearby.

If you are pursuing graduate education, carefully examine the courses offered. Some programs are organized around human development and human conflicts, which are psychodynamic concepts; other programs are not.

The American Psychoanalytic Association (www.apsa.org), American Psychological Association (www.apa.org), International Psychoanalytic Association (www.IPA.world), American Psychiatric Association (www.psychiatry.org), and local psychoanalytic institutes and organizations all provide continuing education courses in psychodynamic psychotherapy.

# ABOUT THE AUTHOR

RONALD L. FUREDY, M.D., is a psychiatrist and psychoanalyst. He was the past director of psychiatry at the University of Washington Harborview Medical Center. During his tenure, the psychiatry residents honored him with the outstanding teaching award. He moved to full-time clinical practice and pursued his psychoanalytic training at the Seattle Psychoanalytic Society and Institute (SPSI), where he is presently a Training and Consulting Analyst emeritus. At SPSI, he was nominated by the psychoanalytic students and received the outstanding teaching award twice. He is a fellow of the American Board of Psychoanalysis. He has devoted over fifty years of his professional life to practicing, studying, and teaching psychodynamic psychotherapy and psychoanalysis for individuals suffering from emotional pain.

Made in United States
North Haven, CT
10 November 2026

22096538R00099